# About this Series

*IDEAS IN PROGRESS* is a commercially published series of working papers dealing with alternatives to industrial society. It is our belief that the ills and frustrations which have overtaken mankind are not merely due to industrial civilization's inadequate planning and faulty execution, but are caused by fundamental errors in our basic thinking about goals. This series is designed to question and rethink the underlying concepts of many of our institutions and to propose alternatives. Unless this is done soon society will undoubtedly create even greater injustices and inequalities than at present. It is to correct this trend that authors are invited to submit short texts of work in progress of interest not only to their colleagues but also to the general public. The series fosters direct contact between the author and the reader. It provides the author with the opportunity to give wide circulation to his draft while he is still developing an idea. It offers the reader an opportunity to participate critically in shaping this idea before it has taken on a definitive form.

Future editions of a paper may include the author's revisions and critical reactions from the public. Readers are invited to write directly to the authors of the present volume at the following addresses:

Mr. Peter Diggory, 10 Campden Hill Square, London W8 7LB
Dr. John McEwan, 193 Camberwell Grove, London SE5 8JU

THE PUBLISHERS

# ABOUT THE AUTHORS

Peter Diggory, married with two children, is senior gynaecologist to the Kingston Group of Hospitals and honorary consultant to the Royal Marsden Hospital. He trained as a physicist and worked on radar research, taking up medicine only in 1946. He has always been interested in the social aspects of his specialty and was adviser to David Steel who sponsored the Abortion Act, 1968. He has served the World Health Organization as consultant in Maternal and Child Health problems in India and Bangladesh. He has written numerous papers in medical journals and is a contributor to *Human Reproduction*, edited by Hafez and Evans (Harper & Row, 1973).

John McEwan, married with two children, is a family doctor in S.E. London and holds a unique post as National Health Service Consultant in Family Planning at King's College Hospital where he has helped to build up a comprehensive service providing contraception, sterilization, and abortion for the local district. He is a teacher of medical students, doctors, and nurses as well as being involved in research projects on contraceptive methods and fertility behaviour.

# PLANNING
## OR
# PREVENTION?

IDEAS IN PROGRESS

# PLANNING
# OR
# PREVENTION?

## THE NEW FACE OF 'FAMILY PLANNING'

Peter Diggory
and
John McEwan

MARION BOYARS · LONDON

**A MARION BOYARS BOOK**
distributed by
Calder & Boyars Ltd
18 Brewer Street, London WIR 4AS
First published in Great Britain in 1976 by
Marion Boyars Publishers Ltd
18 Brewer Street, London WIR 4AS

ISBN 0-7145-2552-9 Cased Edition
ISBN 0-7145-2553-7 Paperback Edition

Printed in Great Britain
by Ebenezer Baylis and Son Limited
The Trinity Press, Worcester, and London

# TABLE OF CONTENTS

# PREFACE

We have prepared this working paper for 'Ideas in Progress', writing as two doctors who have a long involvement in Family Planning. We shall explain why we do not equate this with population control and why in our view clinicians should not become directly involved in the latter. We have attempted to present the evidence and arguments objectively. We admit that we have axes to grind, but we do try to describe human behaviour without casting any judgment.

Doctors are concerned with their patients as individuals with problems, but in the realm of Family Planning the relationship is more that of adviser and client, and the doctor's role is supportive. We are paternalistic because of our training and practice in clinical medicine: our day-to-day lives involve decisions about individuals and their specific problems. In other words we are clinical atomists as well as being products of the socio-cultural pattern of our times. Both of us have also been concerned with aspects of legal and administrative reform in Family Planning Services; and even with medical services outside the U.K. related to population control, and we see very clearly the inadequacies of such services to the personal problems of our clients. We have tried always to take a client-centred view of the moral and political aspects of the issues at stake.

Neither of us is religious in the denominational sense, though we are reluctant to accept labels such as humanist, agnostic, or atheist since these terms may not be appropriate to the attitudes we take up. While not denying a central place to the spiritual life, we think that the extreme manifestations of denominational religion interfere with the sexual and psychological equilibria we are trying to promote in the cause of health.

Our initial training as doctors was in the natural sciences and on this basis we had to acquire competence in the wide-ranging and constantly changing work of the practising physician, in which the strict intellectual disciplines of the natural sciences

9

apply only very loosely. We gain comfort from observing the essentially polemical nature of all the social sciences. The application of social science to clinical medicine is relatively new, and the consequence still uncertain. Polemicism is new in clinical medicine and not without danger for professional men like ourselves who could be loosely described as 'progressive' or individually liberating. In the field of reproductive behaviour we believe that people need to be free to make their own choices, which become more complicated and more divorced from instinctual behaviour with the advance of civilization. We are aware too of the danger of holistic attitudes and of large scale manipulation of society described and condemned by Popper,* attempts at which come both from reactionary elements and from revisionists of the left. Both camps can boast sociologists, or social engineers, whose studies yield conclusions compatible with their own social policies; but both are inimical to our own standpoint. The reader expecting a case for radical and rigid reforms will be disappointed.

Until now medicine has contributed more to death control than to birth control and we are aware of the ecological disasters that uncontrolled fertility could bring. We believe that all healthy societies, especially where the individual members have ready access to the technology of birth control, achieve reproductive stability and that attempts to impose solutions from above are unnecessary and counter-productive. There is already enough demography from non-demographers to deter us from emulating them. We do not pretend to understand causal mechanisms in broad fertility trends, but we do know something of how a person or family reacts to biological pressures. We see fertility control methods and their provision as primarily the means to help individuals, families, and perhaps communities towards a higher state of health in the sense of achieving better physical, mental and social balance with the environment. Birth control initially requires doctors as technicians, guides, counsellors, and educators in the field of human reproductive behaviour. We can hope to be successful only by facilitating freedom of choice and by avoiding doctrinaire solutions; and this is central to everything we write.

* POPPER, K. R. (1961). *The Poverty of Historicism.* 2nd. Edit. Routledge and Kegan Paul, London.

# 1 'FAMILY PLANNING' AND MEDICINE

'FAMILY Planning' started as a euphemism for birth control which was thought too unpleasant a subject to be named openly. Later the International Planned Parenthood Federation and the British Family Planning Association paid lip service to the idea of helping married couples with problems of infertility as well as contraception. In practice neither of these bodies has ever devoted even 1% of its resources to pro-fertility work because they considered the restriction of excessive and undesired fertility to be a more urgent, important and cost-effective task.

Semantic confusion persists, the whole subject being still a highly emotive one. 'Family Planning' is not usually considered to include the treatment of infertility—though this is clearly implied by the title. It is held to include the provision of contraception to the married or unmarried who want no family at all. In recent years, in other words, it has come to be synonymous with 'birth control' or more accurately 'birth prevention' in the widest sense, including contraception, female and male sterilization, and even the termination of unwanted pregnancies.

'Family Planning' implies an element of medical care. In April 1974, the British Secretary of State for Social Services implemented the command of Parliament to 'make all arrangements . . . for the giving of advice on contraception . . .' as part of the newly organized National Health Service. Long before this medicine had accepted some responsibility for the development of fertility-regulating mechanisms. But how successful can they be? How have the involvement of doctors in and their attitudes to fertility control affected its efficiency and the popularity or otherwise of 'Family Planning'?

## The Development of Doctors' Attitudes

Only 107 years ago the *British Medical Journal* attacked the stance favourable to contraception taken up by Bertrand Russell's father, Lord Amberley, in the following words: 'Our profession will repudiate with indignation and disgust such functions as these gentlemen wish to assign it.' In the same year, the annual meeting of the British Medical Association heard a Dr. Beatty attack 'the beastly contrivances and the filthy expedients for the prevention of conception'.[1]

Dr. Alex Comfort has described the ways in which doctors tend to make the public thoroughly fearful in sexual matters.[2] Moreover, the introduction of new contraceptive methods is hedged about with restrictions by the drug safety organizations in the United States and, to a lesser degree, in Britain, so that drug companies are nowadays reluctant to develop a new and promising compound owing to the enormous expense of conforming to the requirements for detailed trials. Nobody wants a contraceptive that produces cancer or foetal abnormalities, and in fact none has ever done so. Such policies virtually prevent the development of new drugs in contraception.

To what extent are doctors necessary to the provision of contraception? They seemed essential in November, 1921, when the Neo-Malthusian League opened its first contraceptive clinic in Walworth, a clinic still flourishing as a centre for advice and teaching. However, Marie Stopes, herself a doctor of philosophy not of medicine, was far from convinced that medical men were needed. Although she did employ some doctors such as the remarkable pioneer Evelyn Fisher, she relied mainly upon midwives both to give advice and to fit appliances.[3] The tradition has been maintained and even today the Marie Stopes Clinic, which remains a clinic of international fame, relies very largely upon para-medical workers. This could easily be extended to other centres and agencies giving contraceptive advice and supplies.

We are just beginning to realize that doctors may *not* be the best people to give advice on contraception. Whether in clinics, hospitals, or their own surgeries, doctors are always in a position of power and authority, and this inhibits just those ill-educated women most in need of advice and help. A group of eminent doctors recently wrote to the medical press: 'We conclude that it would be a responsible and constructive step forward in medical practice to widen the range of those empowered to dispense oral contraceptives to include state registered nurses, midwives and health visitors who have had some additional training in contraceptive practice.'[4]

Bone's study in 1970 of the use of family planning services in England and Wales outlines some of the difficulties she found people had experienced in discussing contraception with doctors.[5] Only one-third of those at risk of unwanted pregnancy took medical advice, and of these most married women preferred asking their general practitioner. Many of those who did not consult a doctor were worried about being embarrassed by the circumstances in which advice might be given and examinations carried out. Medical family planning experts differ as to whether a vaginal examination is an essential routine for patients taking the pill. Only 25% of those taking advice from a family doctor were so examined according to the survey, but virtually all those using clinics. For single women the greatest deterrent to seeking medical help was the fear of being snubbed or embarrassed by G.P.s unwilling to give advice to the unmarried. Such fears might be groundless but they could not know this beforehand. Many single women believed that they would be snubbed even in regular family planning clinics, and for this reason preferred to go to clinics specially set up for them, such as those run by the Brook Advisory Centres.

*Table 1*

| Proposed client | Percentage of G.P.s who would introduce discussion of birth control | |
| --- | --- | --- |
| | *1967–8* | *1970–1* |
| A married woman with 3 children and only one bedroom | 55 | 71 |
| A married woman with 3 children and no social or health problems | 21 | 34 |
| An unmarried woman who had had a baby | 51 | 73 |
| Number of doctors (=100%) | 531 | 601 |

From Cartwright and Waite (1972)

Cartwright and Waite reported on the attitudes of doctors, mostly G.P.s, giving advice to parents of new babies in 1967–8 and again in 1970–1.[6, 7] There was certainly a marked change in doctor attitudes during that time though not a complete *volte face* (Table 1).

One should look at the proportion who would not open the subject of birth control at all. These doctors evidently have difficulty in communicating in an area where commonsense would suggest the need.

François Lafitte in his report for the Family Planning Association, defined a family planning clinic as 'a device for bringing the public in touch with doctors willing to give family planning advice in circumstances where the medical profession as a whole does not regard this as one of its functions'.[8] The report went on to recommend a network of clinics to be set up by this voluntary charitable association to serve the needs of the whole British population. Broadly his advice was accepted and a new system was set up in 1965–6, later to be taken over piecemeal and in part by the local authorities under the National Health Service (Family Planning) Act 1967. Now in 1976 all these clinics are in process of being absorbed in turn by the Area Health Authorities of the reorganized National Health Service.

Clinics have unfortunate side effects: they relieve the ordinary doctor from the necessity of providing contraception as part of the normal medical service; by collecting together people who want this particular service in one place at set times they identify the users, some of whom may thus be embarrassed and inhibited from further attendance; and thirdly, the doctors and nurses working in them tend to make a new medical specialty. This can limit the availability of medical contraception at a time when it should be increased.

Specialized clinics call for doctors and nurses, whom it may be possible to provide for minority needs (e.g. tuberculosis or anti-smoking), but not when the 5 million or more couples at risk of undesired conception are involved. This would be so even if most of the clinical decisions were to be taken by nurses.

Medically supervised contraception, if it is to be universal, must be integrated with other health services. Family medicine and gynaecology would bear the main work load. Contra-

14

ception is then more likely to be acceptable to everyone and to become a normal part of everyday life instead of the minority activity Margaret Bone found it to be in 1970.[5]

## Medical Opposition to Contraception

Now that medically supervised contraception is to become a part of the National Health Service it may be useful to review the long conflict of opinion amongst doctors on the topic. The history of the struggle has been admirably documented and described by Himes,[9] by Wood and Suitters,[1] and by Fryer.[10] The fight has often been vicious and we see its remnant in the conflict about induced abortion that continues today.

Drysdale described simple contraceptive methods in an 1854 pamphlet on population. This followed up Place's restatement in the 1830s of Malthusian ideas on the need for population control. In 1887 Dr. H. Arthur Allbutt was struck off the Medical Register not simply for having written and published the *Wife's Handbook*, but for having sold it for a mere sixpence a copy, thus putting it into the hands of the working class.

Among the anxiety-makers Dr. C. H. Routh seems to have been a kind of self-appointed Victorian vigilante. Writing in 1878 he called the use of birth control methods by women 'sexual fraudulency and conjugal onanism' and warns of 'death or severe illness from acute and chronic metritis, leucorrhoea, menorrhagia and haematocoele, histeralgia (*sic*) and hyperaesthesia of the generative organs, cancer in an aggravated form,' etc., etc. Sterility, of course, was inevitable but 'mania, leading to suicide and the most repulsive nymphomania are induced'. Men suffered general nervous prostration, mental decay, loss of memory, intense cardiac palpitations, mania and conditions leading to suicide'. It is interesting that suicide should be an end result in both cases, but it is noticeable that the men did not get anything analogous to the 'repulsive nymphomania' of the women; perhaps they had it already. Dr. Routh said later in his exposition: '. . . as medical men we are often the guardians of female virtue'.

These statements clearly represented fantasies in the mind of the author, and they probably struck a corresponding chord in the minds of his readers. Anxiety about the effects contraception might have upon sexual behaviour loomed larger than any objection to birth limitation as such. It seems that pregnancy was seen as a proper sanction against sexual indulgence purely for physical pleasure. Female 'virtue' was to be preserved by fear of pregnancy.

How many similar attitudes survive?—Very few, at any rate in the form of such self-indulgent fantasy-mongering. Modern commentators are more sophisticated and aware of possible criticisms than the psychologically naïve and pre-Freudian Routh. But many doctors still disapprove of the enjoyment of sex, and so they criticize contraceptive techniques which they may believe make illicit sex more readily possible. A recent lecture by a consultant physician to a group of doctors on a family planning course was accompanied by a number of slides showing severe and rare pathological conditions which theoretically *could* occur in patients on the pill. In fact, none of those shown had occurred in this way; they were from other sick people. There were diagrams of clotting factors and biochemical reactions emphasizing abnormal pathways in body chemistry, all of which were enough to cause considerable anxiety to a G.P. prescribing contraceptive pills. Yet the serious complications of pill medication are excessively rare. It is one of the safest and best documented drugs used in medicine, much safer than aspirin or many of the pain killers sold over the counter in a chemist's shop.

Medical attitudes towards young people are revealing. Nearly everyone with expert knowledge agrees that pregnancy in young teenagers is more dangerous for mother and baby than in older women, and that having babies at that age is unlikely to be socially successful. Yet there is absolute resistance by many doctors to giving contraceptives to young single people. It is seen as 'opening the floodgates of permissiveness', whatever that might really mean. At any one time there has always been a proportion of young people having active sexual relationships. It is no more than a biological phenomenon, whatever older people may think socially or morally. Mayhew in 1851 described young-love-relationships among costermongers in central London: 'Unions take place when the lad is about 14. Two or three out of 100 have their female helpmates at that early age; but the female is generally a couple of years older than her partner. Nearly all the costermongers form such alliances as I have described, when both parties are under twenty.'[11] Sexual relationships have always been about as common as this in young teenagers.

The difference between the mid-19th century and today is in the behaviour of upper-class girls. Virginity at marriage was once essential, and marriages were contracted in many of the more affluent families for economic rather than emotional reasons. Nowadays, this is less common and many girls of all social classes are sexually active before marriage, which was formerly true only of men. The attitude of those doctors who refuse medical contraception to single girls is as unscientific and biased as Dr. Routh's condemnation of all birth control practices in mid-Victorian times.

There are other ways in which doctors' attitudes have held back the general availability of fertility control. One illustration is the regional variation in the availability of induced abortion in the National Health Service revealed by Cartwright in her study for the Lane Committee in 1972.[12] There were some Hospital Regions at that time where it was virtually impossible for a woman with an unwanted pregnancy to obtain a N.H.S. abortion unless there was a very serious organic illness. These included Birmingham, Sheffield, and Liverpool. The attitudes of doctors towards contraception were more reserved in these areas also, so that there were urban islands with a higher than average frequency of high-parity births and a higher proportion of private-sector abortions.

Another example of the strange attitudes of some doctors, who are out of tune with social change, occurred in relation to vasectomy. Before 1965, most surgeons believed contraceptive vasectomy to be illegal. It never has been, but it needed a national campaign by the Simon Trust before the method gained acceptance.[13]

A special feature of medical work in fertility regulation is that healthy and not sick people are involved. There are no symptoms to relieve, no threats to life or limb to be assessed and countered. A similar situation faces doctors in screening clinics, where there can, however, be an anxiety-inducing process—a 'Tut-tutting', say, over marginally abnormal laboratory tests in an apparently healthy person. Why do doctors seem to relish this kind of thing? —Perhaps because they feel their role and identity to be threatened when the doctor-patient relationship is missing.

17

There is something more in the case of fertility control. The doctor is providing a means by which people may be free to express their sexuality joyfully without the threat of unwanted pregnancy. It has been suggested that doctors are used to the backlash of 'Nature defied by Science' and may feel that a price has to be paid for this freedom from biological constraint. Alternatively there may be a disturbance within the personalities of doctors related to their *unconscious* original motivation towards medicine. To some extent doctors are inevitably *voyeurs*. This can lead to guilt feelings and conflict when the medical care involves sexuality or patterns of sexual behaviour in the patient. Unless doctors are able to understand themselves in this situation, it is all too easy for them to develop a high level of anxious tension, which they then unload onto their patient. Medical training has so far been sadly deficient in providing skills for dealing with problems of sexual behaviour, but it would seem that here is a good rationale for providing it. There is also a general need to include training in awareness of problems that may arise in the interaction between doctor and patient. Balint and his colleagues of the Tavistock Centre pioneered such work.[14]

The form of doctors' future involvement in fertility control is not at all certain. Much depends on the nature of the methods used and their biological effects. Physico-chemical solutions to the problems of fertility regulation are not enough. They will have to be accompanied by efforts involving the behavioural sciences if doctors and all other health care professionals are to make the most valuable possible—and psychologically the least-cluttered contribution to the control of human fertility.

## Sociological and 'Political' Aspects

The discussion so far has involved clinicians—doctors who deal with *individual* persons. We shall now consider briefly the more recent role of doctors in manipulating human behaviour on a large scale, that is, promoting fertility control for reasons of 'social engineering'.

Swings in fertility have always aroused deep feeling and loud comment from politicians and others concerned with the community at large. In times of decline there may be anxiety about reduced consumer markets, a reduced labour force, fewer soldiers to fight or simply a reduction in national prestige due to a decline in national numbers. In times of increase—and we witnessed this in Britain during the 1960s—there has been anxiety about declining resources, and therefore a general lowering of living standards. These arguments have become more cogent since the development of the modern welfare state.

A world problem of over-population was first recognized after the Second World War. Since then many attempts have been made to quantify the problem, and a great deal of energy and money has been spent by the Western countries on the problem of over-population in less-developed areas. Doctors have played a prominent part in promoting such activities.

It is certainly true that knowledge of the size and composition of a population and its variation is essential to epidemiologists in measuring the spread of harmful conditions of any kind and in assessing the need for health care. But what of the proposal to modify population size by medical intervention as part of a deliberate policy?

The involvement of doctors seems to arise in two ways: firstly, the means of fertility regulation involve technical aspects of medical care—operations, drugs, and appliances to be fitted inside the body; secondly, doctors assess the effects on health of hyper-fertility. Sir Dugald Baird gave an outstanding example of successful intervention in this field. He was able as a clinician to introduce a liberal policy of abortion, sterilization, and contraception within an area around Aberdeen in the 1930s and 1940s and, blessed with a relatively stable population, he was then able to measure the improvements in health and obstetric outcome that resulted.[15] The improvement over conditions in the geographically adjacent but less progressive areas was dramatic. Family Planning is now included by the World Health Organization within its maternal and child-health activities rather than as a part of population-control.

What we feel to be a more doubtful rationale is manipulation of population dynamics. There are many pressures on intelligent people to accept this approach and local medical policy has often been based on it alone, but there is the inevitable implication that the policy might be reversed if the population trend changed or if the political assessment altered. Such a reversal has actually occurred in Rumania. In this Marxist country social engineering

19

is an article of faith. After the Second World War there had been a long period of abortion on demand, used as the main method of birth control. So successful was this policy that the Rumanian birth-rate fell and the government, converted to a pro-natalist policy, revoked the legislation allowing abortion. For a short while the new policy was successful and the birth-rate rose, but within a few years it had fallen back to about its original level.[16]

It seems certain that illegal abortion has replaced abortion previously done openly, and it is likely that infection and physical damage to the women concerned is much higher. Perhaps this conveys the moral that a community or nation can react as an organism, and adaptation to change allows any strong fertility trend to continue.

Doctors, whether epidemiologists advising on medical planning, or gynaecologists doing operations, should not base their policies on population dynamics. To do so means that people are treated as dependent helots, not fit to choose for themselves, and implies that population dynamics can be engineered. Instead more should be done to examine the economic causes of hyperfertility in the countries where it is causing concern.

Doctors, being high in the social ladder, are likely to side with those social managers in politics of either extreme who believe in manipulating society in the same way as doctors believe in manipulating disease factors. In the field of fertility they need to look again at the individual needs of people in families and in sexual relationships to find a more enduringly humane and well-validated approach to solving the problems of fertility.

# References

1. Wood, C., and Suitters B., *The Fight for Acceptance*, pp. 143–45. Medical and Technical Press, Aylesbury, 1970.
2. Comfort, A., *The Anxiety Makers*. Nelson, London, 1967.
3. Parkes, A., and King, D., *Journal of Biosocial Science*, 6, 169, 1974.
4. Letter in *British Medical Journal*, 19 October 1974.
5. Bone, M., *Family Planning Services in England and Wales*. Her Majesty's Stationery Office, London, 1973.
6. Cartwright, A., *Parents and Family Planning Services*. Routledge and Kegan Paul, London, 1970.
7. Cartwright, A., and Waite, M., *Journal of the Royal College of General Practitioners*, 22, Supplement 2, p. 12, 1972.
8. Lafitte, F., *Family Planning in the Sixties*. Family Planning Association (mimeo), London.
9. Himes, N., *The Medical History of Contraception*. Allen and Unwin, London, 1936.
10. Fryer, P., *The Birth Controllers*, Secker & Warburg, London, 1965.
11. Mayhew, H., *London Labour and the London Poor*. 1, 492. Mayhew, London, 1851.
12. Cartwright, A., and Waite, M., *Journal of the Royal College of General Practitioners*, 22, Supplement No. 1, 1972.
13. Jackson, L. N., Hanley, H., and Baird, D., *Vasectomy: Follow-Up of 1000 Cases*. Casey, Cambridge, 1969.
14. Balint, M., *The Doctor, His Patient and the Illness*. Pitman, London, 1957. *See also:* Courtenay, M., *Sexual Discord in Marriage*. Tavistock, London, 1968.
15. Baird, D., *Journal of Biosocial Science*, 7, 77–97, 1975.
16. Johnson, S., *The Population Problem*, pp. 126–28. David and Charles, Newton Abbot, Devon, 1973. (Quoting: *Studies in Family Planning*. Population Council, New York, 1971.)

# 2 ABORTION

## Biological Aspects

AN abortion occurs when a pregnant woman loses her foetus before it can survive as a separate individual. The abortion may be spontaneous (i.e. due to natural causes, commonly known as a 'miscarriage'), or it may be deliberately induced, legally or illegally.

Spontaneous abortion is very common. Among pregnancies that have established themselves and inhibited menstruation (so that the woman knows herself to be pregnant) a spontaneous abortion rate of 10–20% is usual. It has recently been shown that there is also a high embryonic wastage in the very early stages of pregnancy before the first missed menstrual period. There are probably at least as many spontaneous abortions as there are pregnancies that carry on to delivery. It is believed that most spontaneous abortions are due to abnormal foetal development so that the birth of an abnormal offspring is averted by the abortion.[1]

An abnormal embryo results either from its inheritance of abnormal genes or from the abnormal development of what was initially a genetically normal fertilized ovum. Abnormal inheritance follows the usual Mendelian laws, and after the birth of an abnormal child chromosomal testing of the parents enables the risk of recurrence to be estimated. Random mutations can occur either in individual developing ova (oocytes) or in the particular sperm that achieved fertilization. As regards the likelihood of such mutations, the age of the woman is of far greater importance than the age of the man because a woman develops her ovaries and all the primary oocytes when she herself is a foetus.* In all she normally has about 400,000 such oocytes at puberty, of which

---

* At five months of intra-uterine development the female foetus has ovaries containing a total of about seven million oocytes, primitive potential ova. At birth these will have been reduced to one million, by puberty to 400,000 and at the menopause only about 1,000 remain.

about one in a thousand will later develop into an ovum. Men do not produce sperm until puberty and the sperms live only a short time.* This means that pregnancy in a thirty-eight-year-old woman involves a $38\frac{1}{2}$-year-old egg, which has been exposed to all the irradiation, drug, or other mutant-producing stimuli ever encountered by the woman, whereas the sperm has existed only for a very short period before fertilization.[2] On the other hand, an initially normal embryo may be subjected to viral, toxic or drug action or to other unknown outside influences that cause it to develop abnormally and thus make it more likely to abort.

Viruses are known to pass the 'placental barrier' so that when the mother is infected her foetus will be too. German measles infection in early pregnancy has been shown to cause numerous serious forms of foetal abnormality, the predominant type being related to the stage of foetal development reached at the time of maternal infection. Cytomegaloviruses are now recognized as an even more common source of foetal infection: approximately one in every hundred babies born in the U.K. can be shown to be excreting this type of virus at the time of birth; and of these between 5% and 15% will show mental retardation in later life.[3] Several other viruses, including those of hepatitis, cold sores, measles, mumps, poliomyelitis and the influenzas are all suspected of causing intra-uterine death and, therefore, spontaneous abortion.† The hepatitis and influenza viruses may be responsible for some congenital deformities, but this has not yet been proved. Serious viral infections, such as smallpox, frequently cause foetal death. On the other hand pregnant women infected with chickenpox give birth to babies similarly infected, but there

* The testicular cells, or stem cells, from which the sperm bud off have existed from embryonic life and are therefore liable to induced chromosomal changes. Such changes, however, are believed to inhibit or prevent the production of sperm by the affected cells. The age of the man is therefore of less importance than that of the woman as regards the danger of mutant effects.

† Since all viruses pass the placental barrier the foetus is always infected in any viral disease of the mother. Many viruses, such as chickenpox, appear to produce only transient and insignificant effects. Rubella, cytomegalovirus and a few others are known to be responsible for the production of foetal abnormalities. They may sometimes cause foetal death. When the foetus dies, from whatever cause, spontaneous abortion normally follows. There are some viruses, such as hepatitis, which are suspected of causing foetal death and possibly causing some foetal abnormalities without killing the foetus, but a great deal more statistical information and research is needed. There may be some viruses that kill without ever causing later abnormalities.

23

has so far been no evidence to suggest that the children are deformed or retarded.

The administration of drugs to the mother may also result in abnormal foetal development. The only important example was the thalidomide disaster. This sedative drug was taken by a large number of pregnant women and in a few cases abnormal babies were born. The number of such deformed babies born was so small that study of world graphs of deformed births would not reveal the years when thalidomide was an active factor. The conscience of society, and of the medical profession in particular, was aroused, and since that time all new drugs have been subjected to stringent testing in animals to try to avert any repetition. A very small number of drugs has now been shown to cause abnormal foetal development and it remains possible that food additives, etc., may still be actively responsible. On the whole it is unlikely that drugs are responsible for more than a very tiny proportion of the large number of deformed babies delivered.

The developing foetus may suffer actual mechanical damage during uterine life. Occasionally constricting fibrous bands occur and obstruct the blood-supply to and thereby the normal development of a limb or some other part of the foetus. Certain orthopaedic deformities such as a congenitally dislocated hip or club foot may be due to abnormal positioning and pressure effects upon the foetus. Despite all these known causes it must be admitted that the majority of foetal abnormalities are inexplicable.

Much research is being carried out in order to develop methods of detecting foetal abnormalities in early pregnancy so that the mother may be offered the choice of an abortion. Immunological tests on the mother's blood can detect rising antibody levels against viral or other infections known to cause foetal abnormality and are used routinely. Such tests are of particular value where the mother has been exposed to German measles early in pregnancy. A direct test of foetal cells and metabolites is possible when the pregnancy has progressed to about the 15th week. By this time the uterus is sufficiently enlarged to allow the introduction of a needle through the abdominal wall into the uterus, and the sampling by withdrawal of a small quantity of the liquor or amniotic fluid surrounding the foetus—a procedure known as amniocentesis. The fluid is examined in two different ways: by cell-culture with chromosomal analysis for congenital abnormality (very important in older women who are more liable to have a mongol baby), and by biochemical investigations designed to show either the presence of abnormal or the absence of normal enzymes, thereby indicating abnormal foetal development. [4]

Because of the small but definite risk to the foetus of amniocentesis it is not performed unless the woman has decided that she would wish to have an abortion if it was shown that her foetus were abnormal. In practice, once the position has been explained and the probable accuracy of the tests discussed, virtually all women at risk ask for the tests to be done and for a subsequent abortion if indicated.

Since foetal abnormality has been recognized as a very important cause of spontaneous abortion, the whole treatment of women threatening to abort has changed. It is now considered essential to try and find the cause of the abortion before initiating elaborate treatment to try and prevent it. Even if a drug were developed capable of preventing all abortions in early pregnancy obstetricians would not use it routinely in case they were saving abnormal foetuses and therefore deformed babies. The present position is that we possess relatively inefficient drugs to inhibit abortion and we have only a few reliable tests for one or two of the common foetal abnormalities. It is to be hoped that our capacity to detect abnormality early in pregnancy progresses more rapidly than our search for an anti-abortion drug.

## Induced Abortion in Fertility Control

Throughout recorded history women with unwanted pregnancies have resorted to induced abortion. The attitude of societies has varied from complete acceptance of abortion to total prohibition, but this has had surprisingly little effect upon the actions of a woman determined to end a pregnancy she did not wish to go on with. As with other aspects of sexual behaviour, there is a great gulf between the professed attitude of society and the actions of its individual members.

Induced abortion is one of the most important factors in the voluntary control of human fertility. In 1973 the world population was estimated to be 3,860 million people with over 130 million births and 54 million deaths per year.[5] The number of abortions is hard to estimate since most of them are illegal and concealed. A reasonably informed guess would suggest about 25 million illegal and 15 million legal abortions annually.[6]

The rapid increase in world population since the early 19th century reflects man's increasing powers of 'death control' achieved mainly by improved control over his environment including improved nutrition, housing, sanitation, and social organization and better disease control. Only very recently indeed has birth control become a factor of significance operating in the opposite direction. In England death-rates began to fall at the beginning of the 19th century. The birth-rate shows a sharp and continuing fall starting about 1878—the year of the Bradlaugh-Besant trial.[7] This date has been accepted by some as the beginning of effective contraceptive use in England, but it must be too early. The contraceptive methods available were too unreliable to account for the dramatic fall in the birth-rate at that time. There is no reasonable alternative to regarding the fall in the English birth-rate occurring in the final quarter of the 19th century as being due primarily to the use of induced abortion. The medical journals of the time were full of reports of the evils of this practice.

In the United Kingdom and other countries the use of both abortion and contraception increased rapidly in the early 20th century, and by the 1930s the widespread recourse to abortion had become a matter of national and international concern. The League of Nations Report suggested that 'abortion is a greater cause of maternal death than is full-term confinement'.[8] In 1939 the British Inter-Departmental Committee on Abortion accepted that criminal abortion was frequent, and that there was a marked rise in its use.[9] The Committee was unable to obtain reliable quantitative data.

The illegal abortion rate in a country is influenced by many factors. For example, in some less developed countries whose culture and economy favour large families there may be little use of any form of birth control; and when people living in them begin to realize the value of restricting family size their first efforts in the use of contraception are likely to be inefficient, and they are therefore likely to resort to induced abortion. Thus the first demographic effect of a people becoming convinced of the benefits of birth control will commonly be an increase in abortion, and only secondarily an efficient use of contraception. India illustrates this well; the Indian Government recently reviewed its elaborate and costly Family Planning Campaign, started in 1952. They concluded that the Campaign had averted 16·3 million births up to January 1974.[10] The official Shah Commission, reporting to the Indian Government in 1969, estimated that there were 3·5 million criminal abortions in India annually. An abortion followed by unprotected intercourse may not protect the woman for a year, but it is obvious that the Indian abortionists avert several times as many births as the whole of the Indian family planning movement.

When passing liberal abortion laws, only the governments of China, Tunisia, and Singapore explicitly gave fertility control as one of the objectives of the legislation. Clearly other countries must have recognized the value of abortion as a back-up to contraception. For example, the Indian Government were well aware of what would happen if they were to prevent the 3·5 million annual criminal abortions without arranging for an equivalent number to be performed legally. Indeed, India does go some way towards recognizing the place of abortion in genuine fertility control because Indian law permits abortion when the unwanted pregnancy is the result of contraceptive failure.

Common sense insists that, when early marriage and rapid family building—both characteristics of the less-developed nations—are the norm, even strongly motivated couples will have contraceptive failures in the many years remaining after they have had as many children as they want. Until sterilization by means, say, of vasectomy can be made available, abortion is essential if there is to be a real chance of people having no more children than they really want.

In countries where family living standards would be adversely affected by extra children, but where religious or other factors mitigate against contraception, the illegal abortion rates are usually very high. France and Italy are both believed to have more criminal abortions than they have births.[11] The Irish Republic would appear to be an exception.

Even in countries where the need for a smaller family size has been widely accepted and where contraceptive use is effective, there will nevertheless always be some unplanned pregnancies, and unless legal abortion is freely available, there will be many

27

criminal abortions. United Kingdom experience illustrates this. The number of illegal abortions before the Abortion Act of 1967 came into force is unknown, but when the Act was being debated in Parliament Mr. Roy Jenkins, then Home Secretary, estimated 100,000 criminal abortions per annum against total births of 800,000 per annum.[12] Currently there are 120,000 abortions on women living in England and Wales, yet the birth-rate has fallen only very slightly since 1968—thanks probably to the more efficient and widespread use of contraception. Unless sexual behaviour altered suddenly and radically at the time the Abortion Act was passed, there is no way of explaining how such a dramatic rise in legal abortion has had such a slight effect upon the birth-rate unless previously there had indeed been a comparable number of criminal abortions.

When considering the statistics of criminal abortion, people easily forget the fear, despair, and misery they represent. The feeling of threat and the anxiety engendered even by facing a minor operation by a known surgeon in a well-equipped hospital is something we can all envisage. The situation accepted by the 35 million women who world-wide submit themselves to illegal abortions under far from ideal conditions each year exceeds this very greatly.

In some European countries and in the U.S.A. before abortion was legalized many of these criminal abortions were performed by doctors, but elsewhere the level of technical training of the criminal abortionist is not high. In the developed countries most criminal abortions are nowadays 'covered' by the administration of antibiotics, usually obtained by relatively minor fraud, or else openly where they are freely available. In the less developed countries, the risks of infection are far higher; and although death may be rare, subsequent chronic pelvic illness is common. Ten years ago, the commonest cause of female sterility in the U.K. was a previously infected criminal abortion. This has undoubtedly decreased but is almost certainly true of many other countries today. It may be acceptable where the woman is already the mother of as many children as she can manage, but it is a great personal tragedy to the young single girl.

Enduring an abortion has proved to be an effective learning experience in developed countries, and is usually followed by improved use of contraception. For the greater part of the world, and particularly where criminal abortion is most common—in South America, for example—the facilities for contraceptive advice and supplies are simply not available. Under such circumstances, repeated and dangerous abortion is widely practised as a standard method of fertility control.

## The Law, Ethics and Religion

Before the turn of the century abortion was illegal throughout the world. By 1972 some 58% of the world's population lived in countries permitting abortion on grounds other than purely medical.[13] In practice, however, there were vast differences in the ways in which these laws were interpreted and abortion utilized. In the United States, abortion is freely available as a woman's right, and costs are relatively low. In the United Kingdom the law is nominally far less liberal and there is, in fact, a good deal of difference between the availability of abortion free of charge within the National Health Service and its availability privately. In India, where the law is more liberal than in the U.K., and where the need is great and criminal abortion rife, the medical profession has remained uninfluenced by legal changes and in 1972 only 72,000 legal abortions were performed.[14] This illustrates the fact that not only must the abortion law be liberal, but the medical leadership of a country must favour therapeutic abortions by doctors rather than force women who cannot tolerate an unwanted pregnancy to a criminal abortionist.

Abortion as a method of family limitation has not gained acceptance, but in practice it is widely used for just this purpose. In the U.S.A. and in the U.K. well over 95% of all abortions are performed on social rather than strictly medical grounds, and so abortion is used in both countries as a method of birth control. This does not mean that abortion is preferred in either country to contraception. Where there is a real choice and the woman has thought out the problem of unwanted pregnancy, contraception is preferred to abortion.

Japan is an example of a country that used abortion deliberately as a prime method of family limitation. Between the years 1948 and 1958 15,000,000 registered abortions were performed in Japan, and only in more recent years has a concerted effort been made to promote contraceptive usage.[15, 16] The Japanese people

29

showed little revulsion towards abortion. Sophisticated and high-principled Japanese women will admit to multiple abortions as freely as American or English women will discuss their contraceptive techniques. The post-war Japanese 'economic miracle' could probably not have been achieved without effective fertility control. Up to now no country has ever managed to achieve without widespread use of abortion the population stability then needed and gained by Japan.

Statistics aside, abortion can be fully understood only at a personal level, whether that of the woman seeking abortion, or that of the doctor to whom she turns for guidance and help. For some abortion is murder; they should neither seek it nor take part in its performance. Doctors in this group should recognize that their patients are entitled to another medical opinion. For those of us who do not regard abortion as murder the main problem should be how to utilize it effectively within the wider field of birth control. In the West this is not how we react in practice; most prefer contraception to abortion. Initially the preference may have been based on the belief that abortion carried medical risks higher than those of effective contraception, and is a traumatic experience. Recent statistics show that the risks of preventing births by taking the pill or by very early out-patient abortion without general anaesthesia are approximately the same.[17] There are large numbers of Russian and Japanese doctors who refuse to use the pill or the intra-uterine device because they consider them too dangerous and regard repeated abortion as being far safer.

Personal attitudes to abortion are rarely logical and rational. Extremists tend to be emotionally committed. On the one hand there are those who for religious or ethical reasons regard abortion as killing an individual human being and who totally eschew induced abortion. Even adherents to this clear-cut moral position usually show some inconsistency, because their position ought to compel them to regard all spontaneous miscarriages as deaths requiring some kind of funeral—which, of course, is not the case. On the other hand, women liberationists, insisting that a doctor perform abortion on demand as a woman's right, tend to hold this right as more important than their right to good medical treatment for some other less emotive condition than pregnancy.

Neither theologians nor doctors can agree on when the life of a distinct person begins. Legally life begins when a separate existence becomes possible, and in Britain this is accepted as the 28th week of menstrual age. Before this the loss of the foetus is abortion; subsequently it is premature birth or stillbirth. With modern neonatal care children born earlier than the 28th week have survived and this forms the basis of the Lane Committee's recommendation that legal induced abortion be restricted to earlier than the 24th week. Most liberal gynaecologists would accept this restriction as reasonable.

Failure to recognize that for effective birth control abortion is an essential back-up to contraception has rendered many national family-planning programmes ineffective. Reasons for this failure are frequently historical. Those first working to promote contraception advocated it both as a family planning measure and as a method of reducing the high rate of illegally induced abortion. In their thinking, therefore, family planners were advocates of contraception and opposed to abortion. When contraception had become socially acceptable and approved, many family planners found themselves still prejudiced against abortion; and so problems arise when a woman presents them with an unwanted pregnancy due to a failure of contraception.

Most Christian churches recognize a difference between contraception and abortion. Nowadays, there is little Christian opposition to contraception, except by the Roman Catholic Church which officially forbids 'artificial' contraception as firmly as it does abortion. This Catholic edict against contraception has almost certainly increased the use of criminal abortion in Catholic countries. In Britain and America, where legal abortion is easily obtained, it has been shown that Catholic women use this facility as readily as their Protestant or agnostic sisters.[18, 19] As with contraception, acceptance of abortion is little influenced by religion. In Catholic countries the situation is very different, the sin of continued contraceptive usage being a bar to confession and absolution. Catholic women for whom the accepted Catholic method use of the safe period does not work, are faced with the alternatives of sexual abstinence, childbearing indefinitely repeated or abortion. Abortion is a sin and it is possible to be contrite and genuinely promise to avoid it in the future. In other words, confession and absolution are available to the woman who has an abortion, even though she may have one repeatedly.

31

There are parts of the world—for example, the Far East and Africa—where cultural factors rather than religion govern the acceptance of contraception or abortion. Basically the Muslim religion is opposed to abortion, but the interdict is not absolute. Libya and recently Bangladesh have reformed their abortion laws, and in practice abortion is easily obtained by those who can afford it throughout the Muslim world.

## Methods of Inducing Abortion

The techniques of abortion vary between those of the lay or criminal abortionist, and those of the medical practitioner. For legal abortion the techniques will vary according to the duration of the pregnancy at the time of operation.

A wide range of medicaments is sold throughout the world, implicitly as abortifacients, though most of them are not really active at all. Cole and his colleagues in 1968 reported on a survey of pharmacies, drug stores, rubber goods shops, and herbalists in Birmingham and London.[20] Nearly all sold preparations either to a woman shopper who said that her period was late and asked for something to bring it on, or to the man who said this was for his girl friend's 'trouble'. The prices charged were so high in relation to the costs of the constituents that advantage was obviously being taken of the desperate need and anxiety of the purchaser. Only one preparation, which contained a small amount of ergometrine, could possibly have been expected to help induce an abortion. Thus the manufacturers and salesmen were safe from the law that makes it an offence 'to supply or procure any *noxious* thing knowing that it is to be used to pro-cure a miscarriage'. Advertising phrases, such as 'will bring swift and blessed relief', referring to goods available by mail order, leave little doubt as to the nature of the market. Such prepara-tions are still being sold, and many women will recount past experiences when they took them and shortly afterwards 'aborted'. The well-known phenomenon of the girl who has had unprotected sex being so worried that her menstrual period is delayed explains most of the cases of 'success', and early spon-taneous abortion at the rate of 10–15% of pregnancies will account for the others. Even in a country with relatively liberal abortion facilities this trade surprisingly continues. It is rampant

32

in many other parts of the world, though in some places relatively effective drugs such as ergometrine and quinine are openly sold as abortifacients.

The lay abortionist is a shadowy figure whose image varies from one culture to another. In Britain before the 1967 Abortion Act the great majority of lay abortionists were women, and recruitment stemmed mostly from a previous personal experience of criminal abortion. Few could be truly described as abortionists since they acted only under exceptional circumstances to help a friend or relative, and invariably used whatever technique had originally been used upon themselves. Woodside showed that, although convicted women abortionists did not conform to any stereotype, nearly all were themselves mothers. Financial gain was rarely an important motive. Fewer lay men practised abortion but those who did were more likely to become 'professionals'. Nevertheless, most men actually charged with abortion were themselves the putative fathers, aborting their wives or lovers.[21] The few who made their living out of abortion did large numbers of operations and usually enlisted remarkably loyal clients who protected them from the police, even when charged themselves.

In the United Kingdom before the 1967 Abortion Act few doctors were involved in illegal abortion. There was a small number of 'fringe' doctors who collaborated with psychiatric colleagues and, upon the latter's recommendations, performed legal abortions. In the U.S.A. this 'quasi-legal' system was used to a much lesser degree, and in America clandestine operations performed by secretive, even masked, doctors have often been described by their clients; the doctors always remaining anonymous and acting through an intermediary. When doctors carried out criminal abortions they used techniques modified from the accepted methods used in legal practice. In the U.S.A. for example, the operation of 'dilatation and curettage' (see p. 37) was commonly performed by the medically qualified criminal abortionist, but using local anaesthesia, or no anaesthesia at all, in place of the general anaesthetic usually given in hospitals.

Lay abortionists have often aimed at starting an abortion which will then inevitably progress in the same way as would spontaneous abortion. They usually schooled their clients to pretend that, if medical aid was later needed, the whole process was spontaneous. When a woman having any kind of abortion is first seen, a gynaecologist may find it impossible to decide whether the abortion is spontaneous or induced. A woman may well maintain that her abortion is natural, even when she knows her life to be in danger; and yet when the foetus is expelled, a rubber catheter or other irrefutable proof of physical interference may be delivered with it.

The commonest method of criminal abortion is the use of an enema syringe. This is filled with a weak solution of soft soap or detergent, the nozzle is introduced into the neck of the uterus, and the solution forced into its cavity. Here it may either kill the foetus or detach the placenta from the wall of the uterus so that the foetus subsequently dies. In either case the uterus later contracts and expels its contents. About four out of every five criminal abortions induced in this way proceed to completion, and the woman endures the whole episode at home without any medical attention. Alternative techniques include the passage of some instrument through the neck of the uterus, varying from the traditional crochet hook to a meat skewer. If sufficient damage occurs, then abortion will follow.

Both these methods are more dangerous than the medical techniques. Either may infect the uterine contents causing abscesses in or around the uterus which may lead on to very severe blood-borne infection and permanent sterility. Alternatively some soap solution or air may be forced into the blood vessels inside the womb and cause death by travelling to the lungs, heart or brain. Severe bleeding is common.

An extremely popular method, often used by midwives, nurses, or other paramedical personnel, is to introduce a rubber or plastic tube (a pre-sterilized plastic catheter is the choice of the sophisticated who know that they can be freely bought in surgical supplies stores) into the uterus by a gentle, clean technique which does not damage either the cervix or the foetus. This foreign body, lying between the foetal amniotic sac and the wall of the uterus, acts as an irritant, and causes the uterus to contract so that abortion follows. The really experienced leave the lower end of the catheter projecting through the cervix, so that it may be removed before a doctor is called should this become necessary.

In technologically advanced countries even the least experienced

34

and least competent lay abortionists will ensure that either they or their clients have already obtained antibiotics which are a considerable protection against infection.

## Medical Methods

In considering methods of legal abortion there is a time when the pregnancy is so early that it cannot be diagnosed with accuracy. The 'morning-after' pill exists and can be given to any woman who tells her doctor that she has, within the previous 48 hours or so, had unprotected intercourse—commonly for example, when a condom has ruptured and no spermicidal jelly was used. Such pills consist of large doses of oestrogen, such as 5 milligrams of ethinyl oestradiol daily for five days, or other oestrogens given in the maximum takeable dosage for five days. The main problems are severe nausea and vomiting and also disturbance of the menstrual cycle which may persist for several months. It is a medication only suitable for an emergency. A day or so after the course of pills has ended uterine bleeding (equivalent to menstruation) usually occurs. In any individual case it is impossible to say that an early pregnancy was aborted, but quite large numbers of women treated in this way have been studied and there are no reports so far of a continuing pregnancy.

Menstrual extraction is the term used to describe very early suction termination of pregnancy, carried out less than fourteen days after the expected first day of the first missed menstrual period. It is performed as a sterile operation under local anaesthesia, or where the woman has already had a child, without the need for any anaesthesia. A narrow tube is inserted into the uterus and the operator's end of the tube is connected to a suction pump or large syringe so that the uterine contents are sucked out. The actual suction time is only a few moments, recovery is rapid, and the woman can resume her normal life within hours but is advised to avoid sex for a few days.

At this stage of pregnancy the diagnosis can very rarely be made with certainty—a routine pregnancy test on the woman's urine would usually be negative. The woman herself may already have had symptoms such that previous experience tells her she is pregnant. Her doctor will not be in a position to make the diagnosis objectively. If menstrual extraction gains wide acceptance, then

35

in many cases it will be performed on women who are not pregnant. Occasionally suction abortion at this very early stage of a pregnancy is unsuccessful, and babies have been born whose mothers originally believed them to have been aborted by menstrual extraction. The bleeding subsequent to the procedure, having been wrongly ascribed to recovery from abortion, in reality was due to a disturbed pregnancy settling down. Nevertheless, the technique is of importance, and its use is certain to spread. It can be performed in the doctor's surgery and requires no anaesthetic at all. It is cheap, generally effective, and very reassuring to the woman, who avoids a prolonged period of uncertainty. In the U.K. the Lane Committee* recommended that the procedure should always be regarded as an abortion, and should therefore be undertaken only in approved premises after all necessary certification.[22] In the U.S.A. and elsewhere in the world, there seems to be no specific legal bar to menstrual extraction, since it is not defined as an abortion, and the technique will undoubtedly find favour with liberal doctors working in countries with restrictive abortion laws. Active research work is continuing to assess the risks of infection and other undesirable consequences; but so far the risks would seem to be very small.

Even when the pregnancy is sufficiently advanced for definite diagnosis—usually when the first missed menstrual period is about fourteen days overdue—the sooner an abortion is done the safer it will be. In calculating the duration of a pregnancy the only fixed point for computation is the first day of the last actual menstrual period. This is normally about a fortnight before ovulation and fertilization occur. Counting from the first day of the last menstrual period, the average duration of pregnancy is forty weeks. In the U.K. the duration of pregnancy is invariably expressed on this basis, and menstrual extraction can be performed up to the end of the sixth week. In the United States pregnancy is often expressed in terms of estimated foetal age, which is two weeks less than menstrual 'age'. We shall use menstrual age throughout our discussion.

Termination of pregnancy up to about the 13th week is feasible

---

* The Lane Committee was a Committee set up to investigate the working of the 1967 Abortion Act, chaired by Mrs. Justice Lane. It reported to Parliament in 1973 and its report is widely recognized as the most authoritative document on abortion in the U.K.

by operating through the vagina, though there are various possible techniques. The traditional method is 'dilatation and curettage'—D & C—performed under general anaesthesia. When the woman has been anaesthetized she is placed on her back on an operating table and her legs are suspended in stirrups allowing the surgeon easy access to the vagina. With full aseptic precautions an instrument (called a speculum) is inserted into the vagina so that the neck of the womb—or cervix—can be easily seen and manipulated. The cervix is grasped with toothed forceps and firmly held. The entrance to the womb is stretched by successively introducing tapered metal rods of gradually increasing diameter. The foetus, placenta, and membranes are then removed by forceps. Any remaining material—usually small pieces of the placenta attached to the uterine wall—is then scraped out with a metal 'spoon' or curette. The further advanced the pregnancy the wider the cervix must be dilated. There is a limit to the extent to which the cervix can be dilated without permanent damage likely to cause spontaneous abortion in the future. If a woman has previously borne a child her cervix can be safely stretched more than would otherwise be possible. She can therefore have a vaginal termination by 'D & C' at a later stage.

Suction termination, or vaginal aspiration, calls for the same initial procedure as a D & C in that the cervical canal is first dilated. A hollow plastic or metal cannula (tube)* is then passed into the uterus and suction applied in the same way as for menstrual extraction. In the operating theatre, this suction is usually produced by means of an electric pump which can produce a negative pressure of nearly one atmosphere, but simple hand suction pumps can be used instead. The vacuum aspiration operation is more quickly completed, and causes less blood loss than a D & C termination.

Stretching of the cervix is painful, and used always to be performed under general anaesthesia, but nowadays a local anaesthetic, injected into or around the cervix to block the pain of the dilatation, enables the abortion to be performed on a 'Day Care' basis with great saving in time and expense to patients and medical

---

* The inventor of the plastic suction tube used in menstrual extraction and in early suction abortions was Harvey Karman of Los Angeles, a-lay psychologist whose lack of formal gynaecological training probably contributed to his successful experimental technique. Hence the term 'Karman catheter'.

services alike. The risks of general anaesthesia are also avoided.

There is much argument about the relative advantages of D & C or suction technique for early abortion, but it tends to shed most light on the training and experience of the protagonists. Beric in Yugoslavia has established that blood loss is less from suction curettage than from the conventional techniques. Most surgeons would agree that suction is preferable when local anaesthesia is used, and is quicker. It is of interest, however, that in Japan, still the country with by far the largest experience of early termination of pregnancy, vacuum aspiration has never become popular and the traditional D & C remains the method of choice.[23]

If the foetus is Rhesus positive and the mother Rhesus negative, some foetal blood cells may enter the mother's circulation during abortion and so she may develop Rhesus antibodies which could threaten a future Rhesus positive foetus—that is, she may develop Rhesus iso-immunization. Many people, including Sir George Godber, until lately Chief Medical Officer to the British Department of Health and Social Security, have argued on theoretical grounds that, since separated tissue and blood tend to be sucked straight into the suction tube, there is less likelihood of foetal blood entering the maternal circulation during suction than during a D & C.[24] Nowadays the routine administration of a protective serum to all Rhesus negative women undergoing abortion means that this theoretical advantage is less significant—at least in technologically advanced countries.

Because there is a limit to the safe dilatation of the cervix and by the 13th week of pregnancy the foetal head is too large to be extracted, the 12th or 13th week is accepted by most gynaecologists as the upper limit for safe one-step vaginal abortion. A few highly experienced surgeons may be prepared to carry out abortion somewhat later by dilating the cervix to the same maximum and then crushing the foetus within the cavity of the uterus with specially designed strong forceps and extracting the crushed foetal tissue piecemeal. The operation is completed by simple currettage or by using the suction currette to make sure that the uterus is completely emptied.

Because of the dangers to the cervix, abortion beyond the 12th or 13th week is usually performed by methods other than those already described, though occasionally it may be justifiable to stretch the cervix well above the safe limit for muscular recovery if the patient is being sterilized at the same time. Under such circumstances vaginal termination of pregnancy up to the 16th or possibly the 18th week of pregnancy can be undertaken, being combined with a laparoscopic or other method of sterilization (see Chap. 4) since a functional cervix will never be needed again—that is, the woman does not want any further pregnancies.

The traditional method of aborting pregnancies too advanced for vaginal termination was by hysterotomy—an abdominal operation, a miniature Caesarian section which leaves a scar in the abdomen and, more important from the viewpoint of future reproductive function, a scar in the uterine wall. The operation can have numerous complications and it has been largely discontinued, though there are still some surgeons who feel that its performance is justified where it is to be combined with sterilization.

For abortion from about the 16th week onwards most modern techniques involve the introduction of a long hypodermic needle or tube under local anaesthesia through the abdominal wall and into the uterus. The amniotic fluid which surrounds the foetus is then withdrawn or allowed to drain out through the needle, and is replaced with a strong solution of urea. In the past, strong solutions of glucose (dextrose) were used, but they often led to intra-uterine infection. Later, a strong saline (salt) solution was used; but this can be dangerous because, if some of it enters the mother's bloodstream, it can damage the brain severely and even cause death. A strong urea solution has not so far been shown to carry any serious risks. This process of amniocentesis and urea replacement, will cause abortion, but often only after a considerable delay, and it is usual also to give an intravenous drip of a synthetic uterine stimulant at the same time. Where abortion is performed in this way, the woman inevitably suffers some pain, but as the gynaecologist need not consider their effect on the foetus, adequate pain relief can be achieved by using strong drugs such as morphine. The performance of a late termination of pregnancy by amniocentesis is far more of an emotional and psychological strain than is an early abortion.

Recently some substances called prostaglandins, which stimulate powerful uterine contractions, have been used to induce late abortions. These compounds have been widely available only since 1972, and in certain respects their use remains controversial. The latest technique is to use urea and prostaglandin in the fluid introduced into the uterus; a technique that renders an intravenous drip unnecessary. Other ways of using prostaglandins are being developed and undoubtedly these substances will have an increasingly important part to play in inducing abortion.

In conclusion, two little-used techniques are worth mentioning. The introduction of irritant intra-uterine pastes—'utus' paste, for instance—through the cervix and into the uterine cavity used to be a well-recognized medical technique for abortion after the 12th week of pregnancy. Modifications of this paste were widely used criminally and indeed one brand of toothpaste which was sold with a peculiarly suitable nozzle was highly popular for this purpose. 'Utus' paste is still exported, in particular to India, in large quantities.

The other method is the use of laminaria tents—tightly packed bundles of dried, sterilized seaweed compressed into firm cylinders about 3 mm. in diameter. They are used by surgeons who wish to dilate the cervix above 12 mm and then perform a curettage of the uterus at more than 13 or 14 weeks of pregnancy. The cervix is first dilated to about 12 mm and into the open canal three or possibly four laminaria tents are packed. These absorb the moisture from the cervix and swell gradually. After 12 hours they have further dilated the cervix, but very slowly so that muscle damage is unlikely. Now that prostaglandins and strong urea solution are available they are rarely used.

Fortunately, as women and doctors are becoming more educated to the need for, and the advantages of, early abortion, these late procedures are becoming relatively rare. They will continue to be required for the very young girl who has concealed her pregnancy, and for the older woman who had thought herself menopausal. Many women whose amniocentesis investigations have shown them to have an abnormal foetus may also by this time need such techniques.

## Complications of Induced Abortion

In the great majority of cases therapeutic abortion is safe and uneventful. Nevertheless, complications can and do occur, and they may be serious, even occasionally fatal. In all countries with liberal abortion laws and where statistics are reasonably reliable, the mortality and morbidity of early abortion are below those of a continuing pregnancy.

The main early complications of abortion are haemorrhage, infection, or physical injury to the uterus or other abdominal organs. They tend to go together. Late complications often follow early complications. For example, severe haemorrhage, if inadequately treated, can cause chronic anaemia. Acute pelvic infection may become chronic and may predispose to persistent pain, vaginal discharge, disorders of menstruation and, if the Fallopian tubes have been infected, permanent sterility. Overstretching of the cervix may result in a permanent dilatation and so to recurrent spontaneous late abortions. Fortunately, this is a condition responding well to surgical treatment—namely the insertion of a Shirodkar stitch around the cervix early in any future pregnancy.

The number of non-fatal complications of abortion varies greatly according to different published reports; but this is due in part to differences in the definition or classification of complications associated with unconscious bias on the part of the observer. It would appear that, in the case of death following abortion, such variations in definition or observer bias would be eliminated; but in fact as the Lane Committee Report pointed out, an association between abortion and the subsequent death of the woman is not always clear cut, and so the notification of death due to therapeutic abortion is sometimes incomplete.

Both the morbidity and mortality of abortion increase with the duration of pregnancy; and abortion is much less safe in older than in younger women. In those under 30 having vaginal termination of pregnancy before the 12th week the annual death-rate in England and Wales in the years 1969–71 was only 2·6 per 100,000 abortions. Undoubtedly it will by now have fallen even lower with increased medical experience of abortion and, as mentioned elsewhere, the dangers from having an abortion are probably no greater than arise from being on the contraceptive pill for a year. It carries less than one-tenth the risk of having a full-term delivery.

It is much harder to give figures relating to residual symptoms as opposed to death. However, the Lane Report and very extensive American studies have suggested complication rates in early

41

abortion far below the levels that even the most enthusiastic supporter of abortion in 1967 would have considered possible.

## Getting a Legal Abortion

In the United States, Russia, China, Japan, and Eastern Europe abortion is freely available as an accepted right of the pregnant woman, but for most of the rest of the world it is available only for medical or medico-social reasons, so that in each individual case there is an element of debate and judgment.

Where one human being sets himself up to judge the needs of another on such a complicated and personal issue, the scene is set for distortion and hypocrisy. Not only will the woman seeking abortion tend to distort her circumstances with exaggerations or lies, but sometimes the doctors adjudicating will likewise conceal any prejudices and phobias they have. On both sides of this dialogue the distortions may as frequently be unconscious as conscious. The truth is that a determined woman in almost any country where such judgment occurs can, by deliberate fabrication or by repeatedly presenting herself to different doctors, finally obtain a legal abortion. She may, however, prefer to obtain an extra-legal abortion rather than submit to such an undignified and degrading course of action. Until very recently large numbers of Swedish women either obtained illegal abortions within their own country or travelled elsewhere to obtain legal abortion rather than face the complicated bureaucratic machinery of the Swedish abortion-law system. In the U.K. availability of abortion under the National Health Service varies very widely from one area of the country to another and thus, especially for the very poor and the ignorant, abortion is only patchily available. For the better informed there are numerous charitable organizations providing abortion at low cost—or free of charge to the really needy. Both in the charitable sector and privately abortion is, in effect, available on request.

## One World

It is often said that the problem and solution of the unwanted pregnancy concerns women only. In fact just as men are involved in the conception they are equally involved in the outcome of the pregnancy.

42

Apart from economic or family-building considerations the wantedness of the conception will depend upon the relationship between the couple. The accidental pregnancy will impose strains upon the relationship questioning the security each partner feels with the other. A man may feel some pride in the occurrence of the pregnancy and be distressed by the woman's unwillingness to continue. On the other hand either may be resentful that the pregnancy forces them to crystallize their relationship into continuance or separation—in each case continuing pregnancy or abortion may be chosen; the decision should ideally be made and accepted by both of them.

The political decision about a community's abortion laws is the concern of both sexes equally and conjointly. It is not the preserve of the Women's Liberation Movement, or of the paternalistic medical profession.

# References

1. Hafez and Evans (editors), *Human Reproduction, 1973*. Harper & Row. Chapter 2, 'Spermatogenesis' by Vicar, O., and Chapter 4, 'Oogenesis and Follicular Growth', by Franchi, L. L., and Baker, T. G.
2. Roberts, C. J., and Lowe, C. R., *Where have all the conceptions gone?* Lancet, 1975, **1**, p. 498.
3. Stern, H., Booth, J. C., Elek, S. D., and Fleck, D. G., *Microbial Causes of Mental Retardation*. Lancet, 1969, **2**, pp. 444–48.
4. Stern, H., and Tucker, S. M., *Prospective Study of Cytomegalovirus infection in Pregnancy*. British Medical Journal 1973, **2**, pp. 269–70.
5. *Demographic Year Book* 1973. United Nations, New York, 1974.
6. Authors' estimate based on:
   (a) *Demographic Year Book 1973*.
   (b) Hall, R. E., *Abortion in a Changing World*. Columbia University Press, New York and London, 1970.
   (c) Moore-Cavar, Emily C., *Internation Inventory of Information on Induced Abortion*. International Institute for the Study of Human Reproduction, Columbia University, 1974.
   (d) Nazer, I. R., *Induced Abortion*. International Planned Parenthood Federation, London, 1972.
   (e) Population Report Series F, Number 1 April 1973. Dept. of Medical and Social Affairs, George Washington University Medical Centre, 2001 S Street, N.W. Washington, D.C., U.S.A.
7. Banks, J. A., *Prosperity and Parenthood*. Routledge, London, 1956.
8. The Epidemiological Report of the League of Nations for 1936.
9. Report of the Inter-Departmental Committee on Abortion. Her Majesty's Stationery Office, 1939.
10. Report of the Indian Delegation to World Health Organization, South-East Asia Region, Review of Contraceptive Practices, Dacca, 1974.
11. Duorlois-Rollier, A-M., *L'Avortement en France*. Librairie Maloine, Paris, 1967.
12. Hansard. **732**, No. 60, 1966 p. 1141.
13. Population Report Series F. Number 1. April 1973. Department of Medicinal and Public Affairs, The George Washington University Medical Centre, 2001 S Street, N.W. Washington D.C. 20009, U.S.A.
14. Report of the Indian Delegation to World Health Organization, South-East Asia Region, Review of Contraceptive Practice, Dacca 1974. W.H.O./SEA/MCH/FP/40, 16th April 1975.
15. Muramatsu, M., *Incidence of Abortion in Japan: Analyses and Results*. International Population Conference, Liège, 1973, **2**, pp. 319–31.
16. Muramatsu, M., *Policy Measures and Social Changes for Fertility Decline in Japan*. Proceedings of World Population Conference, Belgrade, 1965, pp. 96–97.
17. Tietze, C., *Mortality with Contraception and Induced Abortion*. Studies in Family Planning, **1**, No. 45, 1969. (September), pp. 6–8.
18. Peel, J., Potts, M., and Diggory, P., in press.
19. Report of the Committee on the Working of the Abortion Act. Vol. III, p. 29. H.M.S.O. Cmnd. 5581, April 1974.
20. Cole, M., Abortifacients for sale. *Abortion in Britain*. Pitman Medical, London, 1966, pp. 43–45.
21. Weir, J. G., 'Lay Abortionists'. *Abortion in Britain*. Pitman Medical, London, 1966.
22. Report of the Committee on the Working of the Abortion Act. Vols. 1, 2, & 3. Her Majesty's Stationery Office, Cmnd. 5579–81, April 1974.
23. Muramatsu, M., *Abortion Research: International Experience*. Chapter 18, The

Japanese Experience, edited by David, Henry P. Lexington Books, C. C. Heath & Co., Lexington, Massachusetts (also Toronto and London), 1974.
24. Godber, Sir George. 'On the State of the Public Health'. The annual report of the Chief Medical Officer of the Department of Health and Social Security for the year 1969. Her Majesty's Stationery Office, 1970, p. 99.

# 3 CONTRACEPTION

THE ideal contraceptive should provide a sure means of preventing pregnancy, be reversible at will and allow normal sexual enjoyment by potentially fertile men and women with no danger to health. Such a contraceptive does not yet exist because the truly effective techniques interfere so much with basic bodily functioning that they necessarily produce side effects, serious or minor, in some of the users.

In order to compare the virtues of different contraceptives and to discuss possible future development it is first essential to summarize the techniques already available.

## Hormonal Contraceptives

The combined oestrogen-progestogen pills are by far the most effective form of contraception. They interfere with the normal physiological processes of reproduction in four different ways: they commonly inhibit ovulation; they prevent the uterine lining from accepting any fertilized egg should ovulation occur; and they interfere with egg or sperm transport in two places—the cervical canal where they inhibit the entry of sperm, and the Fallopian tubes where they inhibit the ascent of the sperm and the descent of the fertilized egg—should one actually be produced.

Such pills inevitably interfere considerably with a woman's physiological system of menstrual control, the normal production of ovarian and pituitary hormones being partially suppressed.

The efficacy of the pill is extremely high—the accidental pregnancy rate when it is taken correctly is as little as 1 in 10,000 per annum. This has meant that women taking the pill enjoy really effective contraception. It has liberated them from unwanted pregnancy while allowing them to enjoy a full sexual life with a security previously enjoyed only by men, or by those women who knew they were sterile.

Taking the pill has certain other marked advantages: the

46

discomforts of the normal menstrual cycle are often cured or relieved; premenstrual tension, which plagues a high proportion of women, painful periods, and heavy menstrual bleeding are all likely to be improved by taking the pill. Most women actually have a greater feeling of well-being when they are taking the combined pills. The menopause is often a time of physical and emotional distress. It is at this time that the amount of oestrogen produced by the ovaries fluctuates and declines. Menopausal symptoms may include hot flushes, hot sweats, emotional instability and often heavy or intermittent uterine bleeding. Oestrogen-progestogen therapy, as provided by the ordinary contraceptive pill, is highly effective in treating these symptoms, and continuing oestrogen administration after the menopause may prevent the bony decalcification with associated backpain that is commonly encountered in elderly women.[1]

There is definite evidence that non-cancerous breast lumps occur less frequently in women who have been on the pill for 2 years or more than in those who have not.[2] The evidence that the pill protects against breast cancer is still very indirect. Breast cancers are commonest in women who have never been pregnant and in those who have a late menopause, namely those women who have had a larger than average number of menstrual periods during their lives. It has been suggested that the pituitary hormones, which control the menstrual cycle, and which also stimulate the breasts, may by repeated stimulation produce breast cancer. Women on the pill are inhibiting the production of such pituitary hormones. It must be stressed, however, that it will necessarily be many years before conclusive evidence on this point is available.[3]

The ordinary effects of the woman's normal sex hormones are maintained by the hormones in the pill, but these may differ slightly in amount and in oestrogen-progestogen ratio from what she is normally producing. In the combined pill oestrogen and progestogen are given together for approximately three weeks with a succeeding gap of about one week, in contrast to the normal menstrual cycle in which oestrogen levels in the blood vary and progesterone (the natural progestogen) appears only between the time of ovulation—mid-cycle—and the next menstrual period. It is perhaps not surprising that some 20–30% of women taking the pill say that they do not feel entirely 'normal', at least initially. A very small minority develop serious side effects such as raised blood pressure, considerable weight gain, migrainous headache, or depression. In addition, there is a minute risk of sudden death due to thrombo-embolism (intra-vascular clotting).[4] Such thrombo-embolic phenomena, even resulting in sudden death, do occur spontaneously in both men and women irrespective of any medication they may be taking. The annual mortality faced by women taking one of the modern pills containing not more than 50 micrograms of oestrogen is of the order of 1 in 100,000, almost the same as the mortality from the spontaneous occurrence of venous thrombo-embolism in women of fertile age.[5]

It is the oestrogen component of the pill alone that is believed to be responsible for the really serious side effects, in particular the thrombo-embolic phenomena. For this reason, the modern pills have an oestrogen content much lower than did the early ones. It has been found, however, that too great a reduction of the oestrogen content results in some risk of an unwanted pregnancy. If the oestrogen component is removed altogether, as in the low dose progestogen-only pill, ovulation may occur, but the other three modes of contraceptive action are retained. Such pills result in a pregnancy rate approximately the same as that associated with the use of intra-uterine devices. One of the main drawbacks of progestogen-only pills is menstrual irregularity: acceptability and continuation rates have been limited by such irregular bleeding. Many women have given up these pills because menstrual irregularity arouses anxiety in the setting of their religion or culture (e.g. Hindu women who are excluded from normal social activities when they are bleeding), though it is possible that the progestogen-only pill in a more advanced form will eventually gain considerable acceptance. They are free from the risks of thrombo-embolism.

Progestogens alone are at present used by injection in several countries in an oily solution from which they are released over a period of at least three months. In parts of Africa, in Hong Kong, Mauritius, and Thailand medroxy-progesterone acetate has been used in this way and appears to be an effective con-traceptive.[6,7] Unfortunately about one-third of the women so treated experience menstrual problems, often with heavy and irregular bleeding, and some have even become severely anaemic

48

as a result. Moreover, after treatment stops ovulation may fail to occur for a long time. This may also happen in a small proportion of women after use of the combined pill. Such failure of ovulation after treatment can readily be remedied in technically advanced countries; but, since careful hormonal monitoring is needed, treatment is less easy in undeveloped countries. Although uncommon, a temporarily irreversible failure of ovulation after contraceptive medication is clearly an adverse effect. It is an effect of the combined pills in less than 0·5% of patients; those with a history of irregular menstruation before going on the pill being probably more at risk.[8]

It should be noted that the oral contraceptive is wholly under the control of the woman and entirely dependent upon her continuing motivation and action. Research has shown the possible feasibility of a contraceptive pill for men. A very small-scale trial has been carried out using two well known compounds combined in a pill taken every day. These are ethinyl oestradiol and methyl testosterone. The former suppresses the pituitary hormones which stimulate the testis; the latter replaces the natural male hormone in the man's bloodstream. In this way his sperm production is stopped but his sexuality preserved. The difficulties in suppressing sperm production lie in the possibility of abnormal spermatozoa occurring during the time of inducing sterility and during recovery. Abnormal spermatozoa, if they are effective at fertilizing eggs, may give rise to abnormal foetuses. This point obviously needs careful exploration, which may take many years. Added to this are the behavioural problems relating to acceptability and regularity of medication.

## The Intra-uterine Device

Intra-uterine devices (I.U.D.s) are reputedly second only to the pill in contraceptive effectiveness. Comparisons are difficult because of the varying characteristics of the people studied, but clinical trials of different devices have shown pregnancy rates not less than 1·5 per 100 woman-years and in some cases four times as high as this.

The advantages of the I.U.D. include the fact that it does not depend upon continuing motivation strong enough to result in some regular action. Once the woman has had such a device fitted, she has to take an active measure, namely arrange for its removal, to restore her normal fertility. Not only is she relieved of the need to take a pill each day, but she no longer requires a continual replenishment of supplies. In Turkey and some other countries it has been shown that the expense of contraceptive supplies adversely affects continuation rates.[9] The I.U.D. remains effective for a long time even if the woman fails to return for check-ups. For people whose lives are not well organized and for those living in poor conditions it may well be the best medical method in spite of the relatively high pregnancy rate and in spite of the possible menstrual effects. I.U.D.s may produce variations in the menstrual cycle, often with inter-menstrual bleeding and occasionally the bleeding is heavy enough to cause iron-deficiency anaemia. This may be a serious drawback if anaemia is common in the community due to malnutrition or chronic tropical infections. Abdominal pain is also occasionally a problem, probably caused by the uterine muscle contracting against the device.

The first widely used intra-uterine device was the Gräfenburg ring, a circular spiral of silver alloy or gold wire.[10] This was regarded with great disfavour by medical teachers from its first use in the 1920s until at least the 1950s. Nevertheless, some pioneers of the method, such as Margaret Jackson of Exeter, England, started using them just after the Second World War for patients in poor circumstances with big families and for the mentally handicapped. She demonstrated relatively good results.[11] Its insertion required stretching of the cervix and this in some hands required the use of a short general anaesthetic. Many authorities considered that the ring should be changed annually with resultant expense and inconvenience. At least one private clinic specializing in the use of the Gräfenburg ring used to advocate that it be changed annually and, in addition, as a guarantee of efficiency that it be changed with curettage should the menstrual period be delayed.

The modern intra-uterine device became possible with the development of plastics capable of being given a pre-stressed shape to which the device will return after being distorted at the time of insertion. The devices can be prepared in shapes corresponding to the uterine cavity and therefore likely to stay there. They are introduced by being first drawn into a thin straight plastic tube, which, thus loaded with the device, is introduced through the cervical canal. The I.U.D. is then pushed out from the tube into the uterine cavity whereupon it resumes its pre-stressed shape. A thin thread or filament at the tail of the device is left projecting from the cervix into the vagina so that by pulling on this thread it can at any time be removed. Dilatation of the cervix is no longer necessary and the insertion of the I.U.D. has been made into an 'office procedure' not requiring anaesthesia. In practice there is a great deal of difference between fitting a device in a woman who has already borne children and one who has never been pregnant and whose cervical canal has never been stretched. Only the modern, small devices are suitable for the latter.

In practice, the pregnancy rate in women using the intra-uterine device, though higher than is associated with use of the pill, appears to have proved largely acceptable. The chief problem has been that women fitted with such devices have sometimes requested their removal because of excessive bleeding or pain due to uterine cramp. Tietze assembled the results from a wide range of centres and showed that over a period of 6 years with Lippes Loop D—the largest and most effective device— 30% of those fitted had discontinued because of bleeding or pain.[12] A further 25% had abandoned the method for other reasons, excluding those who wished to become pregnant. This high discontinuation rate because of side effects has unfortunately been a world-wide feature of using I.U.D.s until now.

Should pregnancy occur with an I.U.D. in place, the chances of spontaneous abortion are slightly increased. If childbirth results there is no evidence to suggest that I.U.D.s cause harm to the baby.

Initially it was felt that the intra-uterine device could be an excellent way of providing reliable contraception in the less developed countries. It is relatively easy to arrange for teams of doctors or paramedical workers to tour countries fitting such devices, and in both India and Taiwan high acceptance rates were rapidly achieved. Unfortunately it is not possible to provide really adequate follow-up and reassurance. A very large propor-tion of initial acceptors asked to have the device removed within a relatively short time. This became widely known and the rate of further acceptances fell.

The mode of action of the intra-uterine device is still uncertain. Davis of Johns Hopkins Medical School, Baltimore, has demonstrated that the surface area of the device in contact with the lining of the uterine cavity is an important factor:[13] the greater the contact area the higher the efficiency. On the other hand, the larger the bulk the higher the incidence of uterine pain and bleeding. These two considerations led to the Dalkon Shield being designed. It has the shape of the uterine cavity in relaxation, the shape of a shield, and was made of thin pliable plastic. In order to prevent inadvertent expulsion, small thin projections pointing outwards and downwards but with blunt feet were present along each side of the shield. The Dalkon Shield was withdrawn recently because the 'tail' of the original model was made of braided nylon, a material that allowed microbes to progress up the channels in the thread and thus into the uterus; and there were reports of infection, particularly in women who had become pregnant while fitted with the device. The shield had a much lower expulsion rate than other devices: removal for bleeding and pain was less common than in the case of the Lippes Loop; and pregnancy rates were equivalent. It seems unfortunate that this device is not being reissued with a different thread.

Just why the extent of surface in contact with the uterine lining should be important in preventing pregnancy is still a matter of debate. The devices become covered in a layer of white blood cells, mostly macrophages, large scavenger cells, and these may be the source of substances such as prostaglandins which interfere with implantation of the fertilized egg.

An alternative technique, pioneered by Zipper in Chile and Tatum of the Population Council, is the use of a small plastic device of a shape designed to be well retained within the uterus but with a small surface area; this small device carrying upon it some anti-fertility agent acting in a specific manner. Pure copper wire has been shown to have such an action: the Copper-T and the Copper-7 devices have greatly increased the utility and versatility of intra-uterine devices as a whole.[14,15] The Copper-7 in particular requires only a very narrow insertion tube, 3 mm. in external diameter, and is therefore particularly suitable for young women who have never been pregnant, and who want or need an alternative to the pill.[16]

The chief disadvantages of the 'active' devices is that they need to be changed when the active agent has been dissolved away. Devices with a copper surface of 200 sq mm can be used for 2–3 years without a decline in effectiveness. Five years is considered the ideal minimum in terms of the convenience and comfort of the user and the economics of the contraceptive services. It is possible that loading with a hormone or similar substance with a very slow release rate may eventually supersede the inclusion of copper. Any such agent used now or in the future must be non-toxic in relation to the very limited extent of its absorption into the woman's system. The loss of copper from current copper devices is mostly via the cervix and vagina—the copper is not directly absorbed; though even if it were, the total average daily amount disappearing from the device is well within the normal rate of intake and output of copper from the bloodstream. It is important that all active agents are also shown to be harmless to the tissues near at hand: the lining of the uterus, or, in case pregnancy occurs, the foetus.

Again, just how the copper works in preventing pregnancy is not known. It probably depends on the copper going very slowly into solution in the uterine secretion. This means that there are dissolved copper ions in the cavity. Possibly, enzymes important in the implantation process are affected by this.

The idea of inserting an intra-uterine contraceptive device immediately after childbirth has great advantages. In less developed countries childbirth provides the only occasion when a woman is likely to be in close contact with the health system, either with a doctor, a nurse, or a paramedical worker such as a village midwife. The widely-open cervix makes insertion very easy, though the softness of the uterine wall at such a time demands that the device should be free of pointed ends or sharp surfaces. If suitable devices are made available, paramedical workers could readily be trained in the simple procedures necessary, and since they normally live in the same locality as the woman they are well placed to provide follow-up care and support. Up to now this procedure has had little success because devices inserted immediately after childbirth tend to be expelled. In advanced countries good results are obtained by fitting the device a few weeks after delivery, but this is beyond the resources and traditions of many developing countries. There is a clear need to design and develop devices capable of being retained in the uterus when inserted after childbirth. A similar argument applies to insertions after induced abortion.

## Barriers and other Methods

The condom, sheath, or French letter is the most important contraceptive method throughout the world. Its use was well known in England before the mid-17th century, and the earliest published description of a condom was in 1564 by Fallopio, the Italian physician, who recommended a linen sheath, moistened with a lotion to be used as a protection against venereal infection.[17] The existence of a Doctor Condom, variously described as physician to King Charles II or to Napoleon's staff, is apocryphal, the name probably derives from the Latin *condus* (a receptacle) as a euphemism for an article already widely known. Even today in common speech 'a contraceptive' usually means a condom.

The primary attraction of the condom is that it is easily obtainable at short notice from non-clinical sources, and can be used without medical supervision. Because of these very factors the medical profession has never valued it properly as a contraceptive. The clinics of the Family Planning Association until recently were staffed by women doctors almost exclusively, whose clients were women. The Association therefore had little experience of the male partner assuming primary responsibility for contraception and greatly under-estimated the importance of the condom, and indeed also of male withdrawal. And now that the medical profession is becoming more interested in and concerned with contraception, the emphasis has switched largely to medically orientated methods, such as the pill and the intra-uterine device.

There are various indications for the use of the condom as the logical contraceptive: vaginal discharge, particularly vaginal trichomoniasis, where there is a likelihood of reinfection by the male until his treatment is complete; a vaginal shape preventing the use of a vaginal diaphragm; when the male has the primary interest in contraception and wishes to retain control of reproduction; premature ejaculation when the condom, by slightly dulling sensation, may be of considerable help. Clearly the unmarried, for whom intercourse may be isolated and not premeditated, may well find the condom a very satisfactory device. The only clinical argument against the use of the condom would be an allergy by either partner to the latex rubber of which it is made or to additive substances.

In assessing the value of the condom, or any other method of contraception, there are two questions to be asked: 'Is it effective when widely used?' (use effectiveness) and: 'If used properly does it really prevent pregnancy?' (method effectiveness). These two considerations are separate, for there may be a contraceptive technique that is efficient but interferes with enjoyment of sex. A couple might then choose an enjoyable but less secure method. For example, abstinence is very effective but world-wide it has low use-effectiveness.

Women reporting an unwanted pregnancy often claim that their partners used a condom but on careful questioning admit that the use was irregular and that they frequently 'took risks'. Many couples use the condom only when the woman considers herself to be in the fertile phase of her cycle, and the resulting pregnancy might well be better blamed on the inefficient use of the rhythm method. The condom tends to blunt sensation, and couples are therefore prompted to 'take a chance' and dispense with its use. For those using the condom regularly and invariably the failure rate is similar to that of the intra-uterine device.[18]

Before the pill or I.U.D. were available, at the time when most of the doctors giving contraceptive advice were women, vaginal barrier methods were the techniques most commonly recommended. The vaginal diaphragm of Mensinga is probably the best known of these.[19] It fits across the vaginal tube diagonally, so that the penis is in one compartment during coitus and the cervix in the other, with a thin layer of rubber between them. It works effectively if a spermicidal cream or foam is spread on both sides of the diaphragm before insertion; and it has to be left in place for some hours after sex until all the spermatozoa in the vagina have certainly been killed.

The cervical cap, looking like a small bowler hat made of rubber, is another barrier, much favoured by Marie Carmichael Stopes in her pioneering birth control clinics in the 1920s and 1930s. Marie Stopes was one of the few propagandists of contraception who stated clearly that it should be used primarily to help a couple enjoy sex without the fear of pregnancy.[20] This

55

is in contrast to the present fashion of recommending it for population control—in the achievement of which contraception alone has never yet been directly shown to be effective.

Female barrier appliances require quite skilful manual techniques for their proper insertion, and for this reason wise contraceptive advisers will try to persuade users to insert the appliance well before sexual arousal. Unfortunately not many do this as a routine. A woman who regularly fits her contraceptive diaphragm but finds her husband inclined to sleep will tend to leave a future fitting to the last moment and may then make a mistake. There is also the need for privacy and washing facilities. This limits the feasibility of such vaginal methods to people living in middle-class comfort. Most users of contraception nowadays expect something more convenient, and vaginal barriers are less frequently chosen. For those who do use them they can be very effective, having accidental pregnancy rates probably of the same order as those of the I.U.D. or condom. As with the condom, most of the pregnancies are due to 'taking a chance' that is failing to use the appliances at a fertile time.

Proper use of the rhythm method or 'safe period' is probably associated with reasonably low failure rates. Unfortunately it requires a good comprehension of the working of the menstrual cycle. Recording of the days in the cycle or of body temperature readings is required as well as abstinence from coitus on the fertile days. Its proper use is practically confined to highly motivated Catholics of above-average intelligence. Even among such couples there will be some unfortunate women for whom the method simply does not work at all. In addition, there is the older woman who has successfully used the safe-period method for many years but with the approach of the menopause an irregularity in her menstrual cycle occurs and she inadvertently becomes pregnant.

The use of withdrawal—coitus interruptus—has been recorded from earliest times. There are few primitive societies where the connection between sex and conception is not recognized. The object in coitus interruptus is to have an enjoyable beginning of coitus, preferably with full satisfaction for the woman, but for the man to withdraw his penis just before he ejaculates. This naturally requires firm intention and a clear mind, and not surprisingly this method can be associated with a relatively high failure rate. Nevertheless, every doctor knows couples who have used the method to plan their family with complete success. Family planning experts have tended to condemn the practice because of the biological frustration involved and over the years all manner of evils have been ascribed to it; but we should be cautious about creating anxiety in others by suggesting dangers that may be merely theoretical. It should be remembered that only a few decades ago the medical establishment roundly condemned all attempts at fertility control in similar terms.

## The Risks of Sex

Of all the contraceptive techniques discussed use of the pill is, apart from sterilization, much the most certain to prevent unwanted pregnancy. What are the risks associated with various family planning procedures? A woman who becomes pregnant in Western countries runs only a very low risk of dying as a result: maternal mortality, the price we pay in mothers' lives for the next generation, is now slightly under 20 per 100,000 live births in the U.K., and this figure includes deaths due to abortion. The mortality for legal abortions in early pregnancy is 2–3 deaths per 100,000 abortions. The mortality for criminal abortions is assumed by Tietze and others to be about 100 deaths per 100,000 abortions, though clearly this is no more than a well-informed guess, and the figure must vary from country to country.[21] Provided with this data, Tietze prepared the following table:

*Table 1*

Annual Rates of Pregnancy and Deaths Associated with Contraception, Pregnancy and Induced Abortion per 100,000 Women of Reproductive Age in Normally Fertile Unions. (After Tietze, Western Countries, 1968).

|  | *Pregnancies* | *Deaths* |
| --- | --- | --- |
| 1. No contraception, no induced abortion | 40,000–60,000 | 8–12 |
| 2. No contraception, all pregnancies aborted out of hospital | 100,000 | 100 |
| 3. Ditto, aborted in hospital | 100,000 | 3 |

57

*Table 1*—cont.

|  | Pregnancies | Deaths |
|---|---|---|
| 4. Highly effective contraception (The pill or I.U.D.) | 100 | 3 |
| 5. Moderately effective contraception, no induced abortion | 11,800–13,000 | 2·5 |
| 6. Ditto, all pregnancies aborted out of hospital | 14,300 | 14·3 |
| 7. Ditto, aborted in hospital | 14,300 | 0·4 |

*Note:*

(1). In 4, the figure for deaths applies to the time when pills containing more than 50 micrograms of oestrogen were regularly prescribed.

(2). In 6 and 7 above, the figure of 14,300 abortions needed to avert up to 13,000 pregnancies takes into account the fact that a woman may need more than one abortion in a year to avoid giving birth.

## Patterns of Contraceptive Choice

The first Marriage Survey of the Population Investigation Committee and Lewis-Faning's Report to the Royal Commission on Population are early examples in Britain of national surveys on birth control.[22, 23] A more comprehensive and informative study is the 1941 Indianapolis Study of Social and Psychological Factors Affecting Fertility.[24] There have been many subsequent studies from various countries, but they are difficult to compare because the sampling techniques differ. Some are concerned only with the married and others only with the unmarried. Peel and Potts, comparing the popularity of methods used by British and American wives in studies conducted in 1959, found the condom to be the most popular method in both countries, withdrawal being the second commonest technique in Britain, the diaphragm occupying this place in America.[25] In both countries withdrawal and use of the safe period played an important part in contraceptive practice.

Peel and Carr carried out a questionnaire survey of contraceptive practices of a national sample of women married in England and Wales in the winter of 1970–71.[26] The women were interviewed one year after marriage and this sample was confined to those previously unmarried under the age of 40. This survey has confirmed the findings of Glass and others of the effect on contraceptive usage of the social class and education of both spouses and of the age of the wife at marriage.[27] It demonstrated that the religion practised has relatively little effect upon contraceptive use. Desired family size (65% of people opted for two children) varied little with social class except that professional, managerial, and white collar husbands were the only groups in which a significant percentage—in their case about 7%—opted for an ideal size of no children at all. Only about 12% felt that the ideal family size was 4 or more children.

As to actual contraceptive practice, it was found that 88% of couples were using contraception when interviewed and a further 8% intended to use it later in marriage. Only 2% were definite that they would never use contraception, 1% were undecided, and 1% gave no answer. It is obvious that, for couples marrying at the present time, contraception has become an accepted feature of marriage.

*Table 2*

Findings of the Contraceptive Practice Study.[28]
Couples married Winter 1970–71, interviewed 1971–72.

*First and latest techniques of all users*

|  | First technique % | latest technique % |
|---|---|---|
| Pill | 54 | 58 |
| Condom | 29 | 25 |
| Other appliance | 3 | 5 |
| Withdrawal | 11 | 9 |
| Other 'natural' | 2 | 1 |
| Other combinations | 1 | 2 |
| Sterilization | 0 | 0 |

Total number of users 1,476

The figures in Table 3 indicate that there has recently been a considerable change in popularity of the various different forms of contraception. The pill has increased in popularity enormously since 1967 when less than a quarter of married couples were using it. The condom has lost ground but remains an important method of birth control, second in popularity only to the pill. By 1971 reliance on withdrawal had decreased dramatically and so had the use of the diaphragm and of the I.U.D. as far as newly married couples were concerned. Table 3 contrasts these 1971 figures with 1967 figures in Woolf's *Family Intentions* and with the 1970 figures in Bone's *Family Planning Services*; but for the two earlier reports the couples interviewed had been married for varying lengths of time.[29, 30]

*Table 3*

Contraceptive Methods Used by Married Couples, England and Wales

|  | (1) | (2) | (3) |
|---|---|---|---|
| *Years of marriage* | 1965–67 | 1966–70 | 1970–71 |
| *Years of interview* | 1967 | 1970 | 1971–72 |
| *Number of users* | 576* | 379 | 1,471 |

From: Woolf,[28] Bone,[29] Peel and Carr.[26]

| *Method(s) of Contraception used* | % | % | % |
|---|---|---|---|
| Pill | 24 | 40 | 58 |
| Condom | 41 | 33 | 25 |
| Diaphragm | 11 | 6 | 2 |
| I.U.D. | — | 3 | 1 |
| Spermicides† | 5 | 6 | 2 |
| Withdrawal | 29 | 13 | 15 |
| Safe Period | 10 | 6 | 3 |
| Abstinence | 3 | 5 | 0 |
| Total‡ | 123 | 112 | 106 |

* Excluding five cases who had been sterilized.

† Including pessaries, douching, jelly/cream, and aerosol foam.

‡ These percentages total more than 100 because some couples reported the simultaneous or alternative use of more than one method of contraception.

The findings of Cartwright and her co-workers also show these trends very clearly. From their studies of samples of married parents of recently-born babies in 1967–68, 1970, and 1973 the following table can be constructed. This also shows the decline in those using no contraception from 16% to 11% over the five year period.

*Table 4*

Present Use of Contraception

| | Mothers interviewed in: | | |
|---|---|---|---|
| | 1967–68 | 1970 | 1973 |
| | % | % | % |
| Pill | 20 | 20 | 44 |
| Condom | 36 | 33 | 23 |
| Diaphragm | 5 | 4 | 2 |
| I.U.D. | 5 | 3 | 6 |
| Spermicides only | 1 | 3 | 1 |
| Withdrawal | 21 | 22 | 8 |
| Safe Period | 6 | 7 | 3 |
| Male Sterilization | 2 | 5 | 3 } 7 |
| Female Sterilization | | | 4 |
| Other | 2 | 1 | 1 |
| None | 16 | 13 | 11 |
| Number of mothers responding (=100%) | 1,477 | 233 | 1,457 |

Some were currently using more than one method.
Samples: Mothers of babies born to married women in the year given in England and Wales.
From: Cartwright, A., *How Many Children*, Routledge & Kegan Paul, London (in press).

*Acceptability*

The two most effective methods of contraception, the contraceptive pill and the intra-uterine device, both involve a remote possibility of adverse side effects. All alternative techniques have their own particular drawbacks. At present the pill, the I.U.D., or vaginal barrier techniques all require the services of a doctor or nurse, and there are large numbers of people even in advanced

61

societies who find it very difficult to seek advice in this sphere from health-care professionals.

Every couple is faced with a wide choice of action with regard to preventing pregnancy, ranging from no action at all to the acceptance by one partner of sterilization. The first essential is to try and discover how important conception is in the individual case. Would the couple be able to accept an accidental pregnancy or would they seek abortion? Linked with this last question is the availability of abortion should it be sought. The woman must next decide whether she can accept the very small risk to her health associated with the more effective contraceptive techniques. Both sexual partners ought to decide whether they are temperamentally able to take contraceptive precautions regularly and reliably before having sex; or whether they are likely to be carried away and to 'take a chance' when sexually aroused. Each couple should decide which partner is best suited to be responsible for contraception, though the decision is again interwoven with whether the preferred technique is male or female centred. Over and above these intellectual considerations are the many irrational constraints on a couple, including possibly the inability to discuss contraception with a doctor or even between themselves.

So deeply is sex bound up with guilt that many people feel that contraception, by allowing sex without risk of pregnancy, interferes with nature and that such interference is bound to provoke a reaction. To enjoy sex without fear of pregnancy is somehow to break the rules of the game. The anxiety is enhanced by the difficulty most people have in appreciating how small are the risks of effective contraception. Here the sensationalist approach of newspapers, television, and the media generally towards reports, even if unsubstantiated, of adverse effects of contraception do nothing to reassure the public. Doctors themselves tend to be basically anxious about scientific advance, and they are all frightened of iatrogenic disease, to which the thalidomide disaster illustrates the communal reaction. That disaster has been responsible for a complete rethink on drug testing. In contrast to iatrogenic disease, if something bad but 'natural' happens to a patient—like a stroke or peritonitis from a burst appendix—both doctor and patient are consoled by the belief that the cause was beyond their control. No such consolation is available for an adverse effect of a medically advised contraceptive.

Since the thalidomide disaster the Food and Drug Administration in the United States and the Committee on Safety of Medicines in the U.K. together with equivalent bodies in other countries have adopted exceedingly stringent rules on tests for all the possible harmful effects of any new drug. All contraceptives are subjected to tests of possible toxicity for the mother, and extensive tests are performed to exclude the possibility of deforming effects upon a possible foetus. The demands currently made are so extreme that drug companies are now reluctant to undertake new developments in the field of contraception. However wise and laudable the intentions of the F.D.A. and similar bodies, their actions have resulted in a general slowing down in the development of new drugs due to the enormous sums of money required for the preliminary testing.[30]

With rare exceptions most important new advances in drug treatments have come from commercial research. This has been particularly true of contraceptives. Today the enormous costs involved in the production and marketing of new substances are such that many potentially worthwhile developments are abandoned at an early stage. It is almost certain that new and more effective contraceptive drugs would have been developed by now were it not for the enormous financial outlay required to meet the stringent testing requirements. The size of this investment makes new developments totally uneconomic for any commercial enterprise unless governments intervene. There is a great difference between the development of therapeutic drugs and of contraceptive agents: development of new drugs active against disease is less of a commercial risk and more likely to be profitable.

For example, in the treatment of children with acute leukaemia, a disease invariably fatal if untreated, modern methods of treatment involve the administration of highly toxic drugs; some of the children die, poisoned by the drugs. Some die of leukaemia, but so long as any survive these drugs are obviously of value.

In Britain the provision of contraceptive advice and supplies free of charge within the National Health Service has now begun. This may presage official interest in family planning developments, but such an interest will obviously extend to cost-effectiveness; and it is at least possible that the Department of Health and Social Security may see abortion and sterilization as more cost-effective than contraception.

## Contraceptives and Morals

There may be more to the problem of resistance to the use of effective contraceptives than individual fear or communal anxiety about adverse effects. Trouble-free, efficient contraception liberates people to express their sexuality without the danger of unwanted pregnancy. The implications of this have yet to be fully realized, but it is quite possible that this kind of freedom can itself produce anxiety, especially where the bulk of present sexual activity is between husbands and their wives. One threat is obvious in a society made up of small nuclear families whose kinship and friendship networks are being eroded by new urban planning: couples are thrown very much upon themselves and are led to believe from the media that their sex lives, given first class contraception, should provide a constant round of mutual ecstasy to be repeated at will for the rest of time. Their disillusionment when this proves not to be the case may be irrational but it is no less strong for that.

Another element is the fear of the moralizers that effective contraception allows people to become wildly promiscuous and to break all the traditional taboos of the patriarchal society. 'Promiscuous' is usually taken to mean having sex with several or even many partners without much emotional involvement. An unspoken corollary of this view is that without contraception the fear of illegitimate pregnancy was and is the real reason for avoiding illicit intercourse, and that morality is not relevant. The propositions such moralists make do not stand up to rational analysis, neither are they supported by the facts. Some people have multiple partners, some do not. Sex without emotion is probably most common in marriages of long-standing.

On the other side of the coin, a recent study of pregnant girls under 17 in the King's Health District of South London showed that the relationships leading to pregnancy were often emotionally deep attachments, whether marital or otherwise, that they lasted for months or years before conception, and that the

64

girls' behaviour could not in any way be described as promiscuous.[31] Most of them knew about contraception but had not used it effectively because they did not know where advice could be obtained, or thought that it was illegal for young teenagers. Some of these pregnancies led to marriage as soon as the girl reached 16. At such a young age the ties of marriage were not necessarily the best outcome, and if pregnancy had not occurred the decision might well have been left for consideration at a more mature age.

In general, older people and those in authoritarian positions have very restrictive attitudes towards sex. Alex Comfort in *The Anxiety Makers* has shown that a similar attitude is characteristic of doctors towards their patients when discussing the subjects of sexuality and fertility.[32] One group fears primarily moral perils, another physical ills. In neither case is the attitude based upon reason or reality. It would seem that professionals and authoritarians in our society tend to regard their clients as subjects of lower intelligence and ability than themselves. Possibly the implied higher status of the professionals is attained only by sublimation of the kind praised by Freud in *Civilisation and its Discontents*: the professionals have subjugated their own sexuality to achieve the status they coveted and now unconsciously envy those who enjoy sexual freedom.[33] This psychological hypothesis cannot be proved but it may explain doctors' dislike of the 'promiscuous'. Those placed in positions of authority—doctors, parents, teachers—may have a problem of unconsciously envying those who are getting a maximum of physical pleasure from their multiple sexual activities, although these in themselves cannot be shown to be socially harmful.

Such speculations may seem far-fetched, but they suggest that professionals and those in authority should examine their feelings and attitudes carefully and develop some awareness of themselves. It is perhaps of special importance that they should use this introspection before pursuing restrictive sexual policies, particularly as far as the dissemination of knowledge is concerned. The most that spreading knowledge of contraception can logically be expected to do is to reduce the number of unwanted pregnancies.

## Social Factors and Effectiveness

In every contraceptive technique there is a 'use-effectiveness' factor which takes into account an element of acceptability:

Use-effectiveness = Method effectiveness minus factors reducing acceptability. Obviously also one should not discount the ready availability of advice and supplies.

In Britain the availability of medical methods in the early 1920s depended largely upon one's education. For the wealthy and educated contraception was readily available, but for the less privileged only a handful of pioneer clinics existed. In 1974 the N.H.S. finally accepted responsibility for providing contraception everywhere, but past failures in the provision of services indicate those groups most likely to find difficulty in obtaining contraceptive advice. Glass in the Marriage Survey of 1965–66 was able to show that among married couples manual workers and wives who had left school early were less likely than others to obtain professional advice on contraception.[27] So were couples of whom one at least was a Catholic. Similar findings were confirmed by Cartwright in a study of married parents in 1968 and again for married couples by Bone in 1970.[34,29] The trend continues though the occupational class differences are lessening. Both surveys show a preference for women to consult women doctors, other things being equal. As with other factors this difference has also declined. A more serious difference found in Bone's survey was that single women—probably the group who seek prevention of pregnancy most eagerly—find great difficulty in consulting their family doctors or in going to the normal contraceptive clinics unless these are specifically and openly advertised for the unmarried. This is probably due to uncertainty about how they will be received due either to the doctor's prejudices or to the possible hostility of the reception staff. Bone's findings provide a powerful argument for the provision of special clinics for young people in all areas for many years to come.

There have been great changes both in total acceptance of and in preferences for contraceptive techniques in the last decade. Now that contraception is to be provided free of charge within the National Health Service faster and greater changes may be expected. Cartwright has clearly shown that the most widely preferred source of contraceptive advice and supply is the family doctor, but until July 1975 there was a positive financial disincentive for family doctors to provide their patients with contraceptive advice. Those who did were not allowed to charge for the service. They could charge for providing a prescription for the pill but naturally they had to cope with any of the rare complications. Now that they are being paid to provide contraceptive advice within the N.H.S. it seems likely that the majority will make proper arrangements to do so; and the use of all 'medical' methods of contraception, particularly the pill and the I.U.D., is likely to increase.

The medical profession as a whole is renowned for its slowness to become involved with fertility control. Not until the passage of the Abortion Act of 1967 did the Royal College of Obstetricians and Gynaecologists show much positive interest in the subject, though there were some notable exceptions. Until very recently most young trainee gynaecologists were advised by their elders 'don't get involved in family planning for if all goes well, you will get no credit; and if an accidental pregnancy occurs, you will be held responsible and be pressurized to intervene'. In recent years there has been some change of heart, but both this College and the new Royal College of General Practitioners have devoted most of their efforts to devising courses of special training leading to extra certification. It would indeed be an admirable thing if all doctors offering contraceptive advice were in fact specifically trained to do so, but it is irrational and invidious to select just this particular branch of general practice and say that it requires an additional certificate (presumably with fees to the Royal Colleges concerned) before it may be practised. It should be remembered that large numbers of highly potent and toxic drugs are introduced into the medical armamentarium regularly, and the ordinary general practitioner is expected to keep himself up-to-date and to use these potent weapons safely. The dangers that could be associated with under-trained family planning advisers are minimal by comparison.

The work of Cartwright and Waite showed great regional differences in the attitudes of family doctors and gynaecologists to contraceptive and abortion services.[35, 36] These differences could be linked with the incidence of high-parity births and of illegitimacy in the areas under study. Waite was also able to demonstrate the influence of social, educational, and religious background upon the attitudes of health visitors and midwives who gave advice on contraception.[37, 38] This implies a need for better training; in an ideal world professional attitudes should not show such correlations. The Royal College of Midwives has recently included contraception in every midwife's training so that they may well be a positive influence in this field in the future.

With the new National Health Service role, the voluntary bodies working in this area will have to change radically. The International Planned Parenthood Federation is rightly pre-occupied with countries needing to develop family planning services. The small amount of clinical work in Britain performed by this organization has been done with the aim of providing training positions for doctors and nurses who will later work overseas. At the moment the Family Planning Association is working for the National Health Service on a contractual basis; but this work is to be phased out during 1976 and thereafter the Association will no longer be necessary in its present form. It has been suggested that it should continue within the field of training, but once the clinical load is shouldered by the National Health Service it would obviously be logical for N.H.S. regional training facilities to develop instead. It seems possible that the active spirits within the F.P.A. will continue working in the field of sex education where society's resistance can still best be tackled by a voluntary body. The Brook Advisory Centres have done much to break down the barriers of hypocrisy and false morality that have inhibited the provision of contraceptive advice to young single people. It seems likely that this organization will continue to attract a clientele. Certainly, now that there is a financial incentive general practitioners may become much more ready to provide for the contraceptive needs of their young and single patients.

Schofield is concerned about the risk of unwanted pregnancy in young people who are having sex for the first few times.[39] He has demonstrated that many fail to take contraceptive precautions at this early stage. Many brides of under 20 are pregnant on their wedding day. Divorce statistics suggest that forced marriages in the young are particularly likely to end in divorce within 5 to 7 years, possibly leaving one or two children with only one parent.

68

It would appear from recent figures that the number of such marriages is at last beginning to fall, presumably because of easier access to abortion. Greater use of 'non-medical' methods of contraception by this group at the time of their first early experience of sex would prevent many unwanted pregnancies and marriages. If condoms were made more easily and cheaply available and if their use were more widely and frankly advocated by advertisements, it could reasonably be expected that some tragedies could be averted.

The ambivalence of social policy towards contraception is very clearly demonstrated by the restriction on the sale of condoms from vending machines. Virtually all local authorities prohibit condom-vending machines in public places under a so-called 'model bye-law' concerned with restricting obscenity. Such vending machines can be found only in the lavatories of pubs, garages, motorway service centres, and very rarely in public conveniences, never in the open streets. Once the barbers', the chemists', and later the pubs are closed, a young man cannot buy a condom. In view of the type of sexual titillation permitted in public advertising such a restriction seems lunatic.

Does it need a doctor, a nurse, a pill, an appliance or a condom to effect contraception? Some of the most interesting of recent sociological studies are those relating to the demography of communities in the past. Wrigley in this country and Henry in France have demonstrated by demographic techniques the operation of conscious fertility control by communities in the 17th century.[40] Undoubtedly one can draw similar conclusions for earlier communities which were conscious of the problem of excessive fertility. Abortion and infanticide are both invoked as explanations. Coitus interruptus, known in this anti-classical age as 'withdrawal' (Schofield quotes a mail-order firm who received a request for a quantity of 'withdrawals') may be the chief mode of family limitation world-wide in more recent times and we should examine reasons for its being preferred even today. Withdrawal requires no drugs or appliances. It does not require consistent motivation or the learning of the technique. However, what it does require is action to be taken at the pitch of sexual excitement. Couples using it must learn to tolerate the act of withdrawal without loss of satisfaction; alternatively, they must accept either a diminished or a non-coital sexual satisfaction.

69

Interruptions in highly instinctive behaviour in animals produce markedly irrelevant activities. Lorenz has shown that removal of the egg during the 'egg-rolling-into-the-nest' procedure of a goose results in what he describes as displacement behaviour.[41] The goose continues with an alternative chain of reflexes—for example casting straw over her shoulder with her bill though it is not the appropriate time for such action. Human beings do not seem to have many instinctive types of behaviour, but the later stages of coitus would seem to be as near as most of us get to such a pattern and theoretically it is possible that deliberately breaking such a chain imposes considerable psychological strain. It is interesting that the latest surveys of contraceptive behaviour in the U.K. show a marked fall in withdrawal as a technique.[26] In parts of the Continent, in particular Czechoslovakia, it remains a very important method. It is almost certain that many unmarried couples in the U.K. use the technique from time to time as a temporary standby. It is also employed intermittently by those practising the rhythm method.

There are special groups within society whose contraceptive efficiency is lower than average. Vulnerable families are usually in poor social circumstances with a larger-than-average number of children and the parents have a low educational standard; their planning tends to be from day to day rather than from week to week and certainly not from year to year, or child to child. For such families domiciliary family planning services have been developed in several areas. Such services are provided through health visitors and a family planning doctor or nurse or both call on the family concerned. The chosen method is provided and demonstrated, if feasible, in the person's own home; but if, for example, an intra-uterine device is to be fitted this is normally done in a clinic. The system is highly expensive in its use of doctors and nurses. Probably an efficient health visitor, supported by transport and a child minder, could manage to take the mother to and from a local clinic or hospital instead. This would make all possible contraceptive facilities available far more economically. Now that family doctors are certain to become actively involved in contraception it is likely that they will prove to be the preferred source of advice. Their involvement, assisted by health visitors, may well avoid the need for domiciliary visits by outside family planners.

The curve relating family size to social class is shaped like a 'U'. In other words, the higher average family sizes occur at both ends of the scale. In many cases at the lower end, as we have seen, pregnancies have not been planned nor have they resulted only in wanted children. At the upper end of the social scale it is more likely that parents with greater financial resources and greater abilities may continue to opt for larger numbers of children for whom they feel able to cope materially, emotionally, and educationally. This choice, sometimes embarked upon rather sentimentally, does need caution in modern times. The psychological burden on the parents, especially the mother, may prove unacceptable when the children are beyond babyhood and she feels like returning to her career—the father, however, being deeply committed to his own work. In ecological terms the children of the rich consume far more than the children of the poor. To whom these resources 'belong' or by whom they are 'provided' is a question of political philosophy.

When it comes to the question of population increase, in Britain there are not many large families, and they are not a significant source of population growth.[42] If we are truly worried about population growth rate, the important factors to consider are the falling age at marriage and at the time of the first pregnancy. Nowadays daughters are born earlier and reproduce earlier. If there is a reproductive pattern in which the first child is born when the mother is 18 and this is contrasted with the pattern where the first child is born to a mother of 27, then over 54 years the first pattern has produced three generations against the second pattern's two. This factor is the main reason for the enormous rate of increase in population in India. Its demographic effect can also be shown in the U.K. when we compare the present situation with that between the two World Wars.

Studies have shown that the average desired family size in England and Wales is very near to that which represents the size for simple replacement of the population. Unfortunately family growth often occurs because of later unwanted pregnancies. It seems that at the present time contraception is not very successful at enabling couples to achieve their desired family size, but tends more to act as a 'fertility holding operation' during the family building phase. After the full family size has been achieved,

71

contraceptive failure is not all that rare in the long, potentially fertile years ahead. This aspect will be discussed in detail when considering the uses of sterilization.

The problem with the more effective contraceptive methods lies in failure of continuity. People give up, or are advised to give up, due to anxiety felt by themselves or their medical attendant, often for no good reason. In a national survey in May 1972, undertaken for the Lane Committee, Cartwright[35] found that 13% of those having a legal abortion had given up taking the pill but most of them had not told their contraceptive adviser of this action, or taken any alternative precautions.[43] She further found that they had no very clear idea why they had behaved in this way, but certainly they had not wished to become pregnant. Is this an unconscious biological urge towards reproduction? Is it that more women than we suspect feel uneasy when taking the pill? Is it that women feel it unfair that they should carry the constant burden of contraceptive action?

There is no doubt that there are deficiencies in the contraceptive methods currently in use, even those that are theoretically highly effective against conception. We need to devote more work and resources to the development of improved and more acceptable methods, and we need to study the reasons why the current methods are being inefficiently utilized. Health workers must be trained to overcome private prejudice or adverse feelings about fertility control measures. Governments, policy makers, and religious and cultural leaders all need to accept the principle of sex without fertility for those who wish it. Finally, those who are growing up need to understand the potentialities and limitations of their sexuality and fertility.

# References

1. Gallagher, J. C., and Nordin, B. E. C., *Frontiers of Hormone Research*, **3**, 150–69. Karger, Basel, 1975.
2. Vessey, M., Doll, R., and Sutton, P., *British Medical Journal*, **3**, 719–24, 1972.
3. Burch, J. C., Byrd, B. F., and Vaughan, W. K., *American Journal of Obstetrics and Gynaecology*, *18*, 778–82, 1974.
4. Doll, R., *Journal of Biosocial Science*, **2**, 367–89, 1970.
5. Vessey, M., and Inman, W., *Journal of Obstetrics and Gynaecology of the British Commonwealth*, **80**, 562, 1973.
6. Dodds, G., *Contraception*, **11**, 15–23, 1975.
7. Pardthaisong, T., McDaniel, E. B., and Gray, R. H., *International Planned Parenthood Federation Medical Bulletin*, **9**, (1) 1–3, 1975.
8. Shearman, R., *Lancet ii*, **64**, 1971. *See also* Kay, C., *Oral Contraceptives and Health*, pp. 73–77, Pitman, London, 1974, for a fuller discussion.
9. Tunçer, M., and Dürmus, Z., in: *Postpartum Family Planning*, edited by Zatuchni, G. I. Population Council, McGraw-Hill, New York, 1970.
10. Gräfenburg, E., *Proceedings of Third Congress of the World League for Sexual Reform*. p. 116. Kegan Paul, London, 1930.
11. Jackson, M., *Intrauterine Contraceptive Devices*. International Congress Series Number 34, pp. 37–40. Excerpta Medica, Amsterdam, 1962.
12. Tietze, C., and Lewit, S., *Studies in Family Planning*. Number 55, Population Council, New York, 1970.
13. Davis, H. J., and Lesinski, J., *Obstetrics and Gynaecology*, **36**, 350–58, 1970.
14. Zipper, J., Medel, M., and Prager, R., *Proceedings of Fourth World Congress on Fertility and Sterility*, edited by Halbrecht, I., p. 380, Jerusalem, 1970.
15. Tatum, H., *Advances in Planned Parenthood*, **7**, 92, 1971.
16. Newton, J., Elias, J., McEwan, J., and Mann, G., *British Medical Journal*, **3**, 447–50, 1974.
17. Fallopius, G. (1564). *De morbo Gallico liber absolutismus*, chp. 89. *See: The History of Contraceptives*, International Planned Parenthood Federation, London, 1967.
18. Peel, J., *The Practitioner*, **202**, 678–79, 1969.
19. Mensinga, W. (1882). *See:* Wood, C., and Suitters, B., *The Fight for Acceptance*, 1970, p. 230. Medical and Technical Press, Aylesbury.
20. Stopes, M. C., *Wise Parenthood*, Putnam, London, 1919.
21. Tietze, C., in: *Abortion Research: International Experience*. Edited by David, H. P., p. 104. Heath, Lexington, Massachusetts, 1974.
22. Rowntree, G., and Pierce, R. M., *Population Studies*, **15**, 3–31, 1961, and *Population Studies*, **15**, 121–60, 1962.
23. Lewis-Faning, E., *Report on Family Limitation*. Royal Commission on Population. Her Majesty's Stationery Office, London, 1949.
24. Whelpton, P. K., and Kiser, C. V. (Editors) (1950 to 1964). *Social and Psychological Factors Affecting Fertility*, Milbank Memorial Fund, New York. For a full discussion of the above three items see: Hawthorn, G., *The Sociology of Fertility*, pp. 40–43. Collier-Macmillan, London, 1970.
25. Peel, J., and Potts, M., *Textbook of Contraceptive Practice*, p. 26. Cambridge University Press, Cambridge, 1969.
26. Peel, J., and Carr, G., *Contraception and Family Design*, Churchill & Livingstone, London, 1975.
27. Glass, D. V. *see:* Langford, C., *Proceedings of Sixth Conference Europe and Near East Region*, p. 26. International Planned Parenthood Federation, London, 1970.
28. Woolf, M., *Family Intentions*, Her Majesty's Stationery Office, London, 1971.

29. Bone, M., *Family Planning Services in England and Wales*, Her Majesty's Stationery Office, London, 1973.
30. Christie, G. A., in: *New Concepts in Contraception* edited by Potts, M., and Wood, C., pp. 143–74. Medical and Technical Press, Oxford, 1972.
31. McEwan, J., Owens, C., and Newton, J., *Journal of Biosocial Science*, **6**, 357–81, 1974.
32. Comfort, A., *The Anxiety Makers*, Nelson, London, 1967.
33. Freud, S. edited by Jones, E. (1950), *Civilization and its Discontents*, Hogarth Press, London.
34. Cartwright, A., *Parents and Family Planning Services*, Routledge and Kegan Paul, London, 1970.
35. Cartwright, A., and Waite, M., *Journal of the Royal College of General Practitioners*, **22**, Supplement No. 1, p. 11, and Supplement No. 2, p. 20, 1972. *See also:* Mitton, R., *Community Medicine*, 8 December issue, 1972.
36. Waite, M., *Consultant Gynaecologists and Abortion*, Birth Control Trust, London, 1974.
37. Waite, M., *Nursing Times*, 12 October issue, pp. 157–59, 1972.
38. Waite, M., *Nursing Times*, 7 December issue, 1972.
39. Schofield, M., *The Sexual Behaviour of Young Adults*, p. 95, Allen Lane, London, 1973.
40. Wrigley, E., in: *Population and Social Change*, edited by Glass, D. V., and Revelle, R., pp. 261–69, 1972. *See also:* Henry, L., in: *Population in History*, edited by Glass, D. V., and Eversley, D. E. C., pp. 448–52, 1965.
41. Lorenz, K., in: *Physiological Mechanisms in Animal Behaviour*, p. 242. Cambridge University Press, Cambridge, 1950.
42. Glass, D. V., *First Report from the Select Committee on Science and Technology* (Chairman Airey Neave, M.P.), p. 189. Her Majesty's Stationery Office, London, 1971.
   *See also:* Ross, C. R., *Report of the Population Panel*, Her Majesty's Stationery Office, London, 1973.
43. *Report of the Committee on the Working of the Abortion Act* (Chairman Mrs. Justice Lane), **3**, 62. Her Majesty's Stationery Office, London, 1974.

# 4 STERILIZATION

## Use of Sterilization

THERE has been and continues to be a rapid increase in the number of married couples who use sterilization rather than conventional contraception. Margaret Bone's National Survey of Family Planning Services in England and Wales showed that in 1970 6% of all married couples relied upon sterilization.[1] In 4% the operation had been deliberately performed upon one or other partner and in 2% it was the incidental result of surgery for some other reason. Bone showed that the use of voluntary sterilization is strongly correlated with family size: 25% of couples with more than four children had accepted it. Usually it was the woman who had been sterilized, in 71% of the series. A further 7% of all couples surveyed were currently considering sterilization: where they already had four children this figure was 21%. Since 1970 vasectomy has become much more widely accepted, so bringing the sexes nearer to equality in this respect and the proportion of married couples of reproductive age who use sterilization nearer to a tenth.

The 1973 National Survey of Family Growth in the United States showed that 20% of all American couples relied upon sterilization.[2] Seventy per cent of these couples had deliberately accepted sterilization and in 30% it was 'incidental'. There is some difference in the pattern of sterilization between black and white couples. Vasectomy was almost as common as female sterilization amongst white couples but had found little acceptance by black men. Over 20% of black women had been sterilized against 14% of white women.

Gynaecological practice differs radically between America and Britain. It is interesting to compare how frequently married couples in the two countries rely upon 'incidental' sterilization; where one or other partner has undergone an operation which has incidentally resulted in sterility. Such operations are exceedingly rare in men and are virtually restricted to cancer of the penis

75

and prostatectomy. The very great majority of cases are where the woman has had a hysterectomy during her reproductive life. The British figure is 2%. In America 20% of all couples rely upon sterilization and in 30% of these the sterility was incidental: viz. 6% of all American women of reproductive age.

Not everyone finds it easy to give up his or her reproductive capacity. Of those who do many already have more children than they intended; and some are couples who have encountered exceptional difficulties or discomforts with contraception. Married women frequently have unwanted pregnancies: in 1973 43% of all legal abortions for U.K. residents were performed upon married women. Three-fifths of these had had two or three previous births, and a further fifth had had four or more. Presumably the majority in these groups had completed their intended family size—a conclusion which is supported by the fact that nearly a quarter were sterilized at the same time as they had their abortion. Most of the sterilizations performed with the abortion were carried out in N.H.S. hospitals, but this may well reflect the fact that the combined operation is inevitably much more expensive than abortion alone, and many of those having private abortions may have refrained from sterilization solely on financial grounds.

The number of unwanted pregnancies is difficult to estimate and abortion figures just indicate a minimum. There are many families, especially those with larger numbers of children where contraceptive methods are not used very effectively. An extra child may not be planned but yet may not be unwelcome particularly in lower working-class families. On the other hand, Bone's study indicated that couples where the husband was in a manual occupation were more likely to use sterilization when their families were complete rather than those in non-manual occupations.

## Puerperal Sterilization

Obstetricians now often offer women sterilization after childbirth. The lead came from Sir Dugald Baird in Aberdeen who began to do so in the 1930s when most gynaecologists would not consider it unless indicated by severe organic illness such as diabetes, tuberculosis, or kidney disease.[3] In most ante-natal clinics today it is a routine consideration for those in their fourth or subsequent pregnancy, and in some centres for those in their second or third. The operation can be performed conveniently and is technically easier within three days of delivery because the uterus is still very bulky and so the Fallopian tubes are still held high in the abdomen and thus readily accessible through a small abdominal incision. It is also convenient for the mother. If in any case she has to stay in hospital for seven to eight days after the confinement, there need be no extra days in hospital for the sterilization—a point of great importance with the current shortage of N.H.S. beds and resources. Sterilization for women at any other time usually entails one or two nights in hospital. For a mother with a full family commitment and a new baby early sterilization after childbirth can therefore be an attractive proposal.

Whether it is a wise time for a permanent procedure such as sterilization is less certain. If the new baby does not survive or develops some abnormality not at first apparent the mother may come to regret her inability to have another child. Similar doubts exist about combining sterilization with abortion. When a woman seeks an abortion she is in an emotional crisis and is not therefore in a fit state to make a decision of lasting importance. Unfortunately the problem is complicated by considerations of cost, convenience, and availability. It is obvious that when a woman is hospitalized for an abortion a further surgical procedure to sterilize her can readily be performed with far less of a drain upon resources of beds and manpower than if it was performed later. In the past some gynaecologists, for motives which appeared punitive, used to insist upon the couple's agreement to sterilization before undertaking an abortion. Such attitudes are now rare. This is partly due to a better understanding of and more sympathetic attitude to women seeking abortion. The other reason is that the usual technique for abortion and sterilization used commonly to be abdominal operation: a hysterotomy—being a miniature Caesarean Section—combined with tying or removing the Fallopian tubes. Nowadays early abortions are more safely terminated by vaginal operations, and when desired laparoscopic sterilization can be carried out at the same time.

## Methods of Female Sterilization

The accepted, traditional methods of female sterilization have involved opening the abdominal cavity (laparotomy) and either dividing and tying the Fallopian tubes, or else totally removing them. The operation is essentially irreversible.

Abdominal sterilizations are major operations requiring general anaesthesia and a stay in hospital of 3 to 7 days. The technique has the advantage that the surgeon can examine the whole of the abdominal cavity and exclude any unsuspected disease at the same time. Nevertheless, such sterilizations require a lot of surgical and nursing time and a hospital bed. It can be several weeks before the woman returns to full health and activity. Abdominal sterilization is now rarely performed unless as an adjunct to some other operation which had already necessitated opening the abdomen. If a gynaecologist has decided to open the abdomen, he is more likely than other surgeons to raise the possibility of concurrent sterilization.

The modern method of female sterilization is by means of a laparoscope—a narrow lighted telescope—introduced into the abdomen through a very small incision. The woman is admitted to hospital and anaesthetized. A needle is then introduced through the abdominal wall and the abdominal cavity blown up with gas—usually carbon dioxide, which is readily absorbed, harmless and allows electro-diathermy and cautery to be used safely. Some surgeons prefer to use nitrous oxide—laughing gas. Whatever gas is used, about 2–3 litres are introduced into the abdominal cavity, and then a small stab wound in the umbilicus (navel) allows the passage of a hollow metal tube through the abdominal wall into the gas-filled space—this tube being large enough to admit the tightly-fitting, lighted telescope (or laparoscope). The abdominal organs are thus made visible and, with suitable positioning of the patient, the uterus, tubes, and ovaries are readily seen. Some expensive laparoscopes are designed to contain their own small operating instruments, such as diathermy forceps. Alternatively, a separate small wound is made to accommodate the diathermy forceps which are visualized through the laparoscope and guided on to the Fallopian tubes, parts of which are then destroyed by heating the forceps electrically. The risks of such operations necessarily include accidental burning of bowel or other organs when the diathermy current is switched on. The method does allow of inspection of a good deal of the abdominal contents, such as the appendix, gall bladder, and lower edge of the liver; but it cannot possibly be as reliable a technique for excluding abdominal disease as a formal laparotomy, which permits the surgeon to inspect and feel the organs directly. At the end of the operation, the instruments are withdrawn, all the gas is allowed to escape, and the two tiny incisions are closed with one suture each, these being removed in two to three days. The great advantage of laparoscopy, is that it can be performed during a hospital stay of only twenty-four hours. Recently the operation has been performed as an out-patient procedure. It is far less traumatic to the patient than opening the abdomen, and complete recovery can be expected within a few days. The disadvantages are the need for a sophisticated instrument which requires careful servicing, and the specialized skill required of the surgeon.

Numerous 'mini-laparotomy' techniques have been developed, particularly for patients operated upon immediately after childbirth. Such techniques usually involve a scar of approximately one inch in length, but they do not permit the inspection of other abdominal organs.

Vaginal sterilization, in which the peritoneal cavity is opened through a small incision in the posterior part of the vaginal roof, is very popular in India where it is held that the vaginal route involves less post-operative pain; and it is not regarded by the patients there with the same apprehension as a procedure involving an abdominal incision. It has great advantages when combined with early termination of pregnancy. The technique requires manual dexterity and a high order of surgical skill; and in the presence of past pelvic infection the operation may prove impossible. It is wise, therefore, that it should take place only where facilities for an alternative laparoscopic or laparotomy sterilization are available.

## Effects in Women

Are there any harmful results to be expected from female sterilization? According to all known anatomical and physiological principles obstruction or removal of the Fallopian tubes should not be damaging. Where the Fallopian tubes have been destroyed or blocked by disease this has usually been unknown to the woman unless she seeks pregnancy. It has never been suggested that such blockages have of themselves been responsible for ill-effects other than sterility.

Unfortunately there are popular myths to the effect that sterilization may reduce sexual interest and responsiveness, and that it may lead to obesity or end up with menstrual malfunction—perhaps because many lay people wrongly associate female sterilization with removal of the ovaries. Many or all of the misfortunes listed may overtake any woman of increasing age whether she is sterilized or not; and the underlying causes may be physical, psychological, or psycho-social.

Muldoon has published a retrospective study of women who have been sterilized and has shown that a large proportion of them has eventually needed hysterectomy.[4] A few gynaecologists have suggested that where there is a need for sterilization, hysterectomy should be the routine procedure since it removes the possibility of future menstrual problems. Such an argument seems fallacious for, although there is a significant proportion of sterilizations performed for medical reasons on women whose ill-health is a contra-indication to further child-bearing, most women undergo sterilization for social reasons as a permanent method of birth control. The first category of women is particularly liable to menstrual problems and, sterilized or not, would be likely candidates for hysterectomy later; but to many women in the second category hysterectomy has the psychological and emotional connotation of a major excision, the removal of an essential part of their being, and is therefore not to be undertaken lightly. Nor is hysterectomy surgically a minor procedure like a tubal ligation or laparoscopic sterilization. So far there has been no properly controlled comparison of the effects of simple sterilization performed on otherwise fit women as regards their subsequent liability to gynaecological problems.

The psychological effects of sterilization in women depend very much on the reason for which it is done and the events in the woman's life leading up to it. For example, those who have had failure of contraception with an unwanted pregnancy or even simply have 'had a scare' may well accept operative sterilization more easily than a woman to whom it has been suggested as a routine method of birth control. Mathematically the chance of surviving the fertile years, after family building is complete, without an unplanned pregnancy is surprisingly low. Since most women achieve their desired family size twenty years before their menopause, even if they thereafter use a 99% efficient contraceptive method they still have a 40% chance of a further pregnancy.[5] The pill is the only method with a theoretical effectiveness near to 100%, and there are few couples who easily accept that the wife should take the pill for 20 years. Elective sterilization is increasingly seen as the rational answer, and it would appear that it is rapidly gaining cultural and psychological acceptance. Cultural backgrounds are crucial to this issue. For example, Nigerian women who accept sterilization in Britain often become depressed with loss of sexual feeling. The cultural background factor to this is that in West Africa fertility is highly prized, and a woman who has lost it is less well regarded as a woman.

Acceptance of sterilization is in some ways like acceptance of highly effective contraception. Once the possibility of getting pregnant is removed the woman is left with coitus exclusively for sexual pleasure. This can make some women feel inadequate, particularly if their background has made them feel inhibited and relatively unresponsive in sexual activity. Sterilization makes the switch from a mixture of reproductiveness and 'sexiness' to just 'sexiness' permanent. Some accept it with relief and alacrity; others feel doubtful and inadequate about their new role. Many of us have been brought up to feel guilty about sexual pleasure for its own sake. Some women are therefore likely to feel guilt once they have eliminated the expiatory possibility of pregnancy.

## Male Sterilization

Do these same factors play a part in the acceptance of male sterilization? Men in Western culture are more conscious of their potency than their fertility. Schofield has described a minority of teenage boys in his sample who seemed to get pleasure from making girls pregnant, but this is not a widespread feature in average adult male behaviour.[6] Dom Moraes has written graphically of the importance of 'machismo' in Latin America to which the fathering of many children makes an important contribution.[7] Fertility potential is also important among West Indian men during the early phase of immigrant culture in London before they have assimilated more of the typical local life-style; more

West Indian men are applying for vasectomy now than five years ago.

The fact that Western men prize potency more than reproductive ability does not imply that they are not such good fathers as others. Feelings for an existing tangible child are utterly different from sexual drive. The connection between sex and parenthood is physiological, not psychological. Many women long for motherhood before it actually comes to them; positive attitudes to fatherhood seem to develop after the event except in men with dynastic ambitions.

Vasectomy for birth control is now an important part of fertility control in Britain and the United States. In the U.K. acceptance of vasectomy is largely due to promotion of it by the Simon Population Trust and its remarkable former secretary, Dr. Lawrence Jackson, who travelled the country ably refuting all the objections to its use.[8] He then brought willing surgeons and men seeking vasectomy into contact with one another. Previously some doctors had thought the operation illegal and others that it was in some way immoral or unprofessional. Now it is a flourishing minor branch of surgery, with probably between 50,000 and 100,000 vasectomies being performed in England and Wales each year. Many vasectomies are performed in private practice, some by vasectomy clinics run by the Family Planning Association or other voluntary organizations, and a few within the National Health Service.

Now that the provision of free vasectomy has been officially accepted as a function of the N.H.S., it is likely that the operation will be performed yet more widely and that it will be more readily accepted throughout the medical profession. One of the difficulties impeding its expansion within the Service itself is that technically it lies within the specialty of the urological surgeons—a group not yet widely interested in social medicine. Most vasectomies performed within the N.H.S. are done 'at the end of the operating list' by general surgeons or their assistants. Family doctors and gynaecologists also perform large numbers, but these tend to be done privately.[9] So far no comprehensive provision for vasectomy has been set up within the N.H.S., and there are still many areas in Britain where the only way to get a vasectomy is to pay private fees.

## The Technique of Vasectomy

The principle is that the vas deferens, which is the tube leading from the testicle to the sperm storage reservoirs in the seminal vesicles, is divided on each side so that thereafter sperm cannot pass from the testicles. As soon as the supplies already within the reservoirs have been used up or degenerated the man becomes sterile. There are some congenital and some infective lesions resulting in obliteration of the vas and men with these are already sterile but will probably be unaware of this until their partners fail to become pregnant.

The operation is easily and quickly performed in out-patient conditions under local anaesthesia. Only where there has been a previous operation, such as a hernia repair which may have scarred the tissues, are technical difficulties likely. Individual surgeons differ in their techniques, but either one mid-line incision or two very small incisions, one on either side, are made in the skin of the scrotum. The vas is identified, freed, and a segment of about two centimetres isolated between ligatures and removed. The cut ends of each vas are usually simply ligated (tied off), but care is taken to try and prevent them coming into contact with one another so as to discourage re-union. This is necessary because in a very small proportion of cases—far less than 1%—there is spontaneous re-union of the cut ends and fertility is thereby restored.

After the operation there is a slight swelling of the scrotum and movement of the testicles may be uncomfortable. Scrotal support by an athletic 'jock-strap' or by wearing a close-fitting pair of underpants is advisable for a few days. Unless the man is employed in strenuous manual work or is very athletic, he can usually resume full activity within a week at most and normally within two days.

Before the man can be assured that the operation is successful and that he is sterile, it is necessary for him to provide two specimens of semen that are found on examination to be free of sperms. Such specimens are normally obtained by masturbation at about 12 and 14–16 weeks after the operation, and if either specimen contains sperms, it is necessary to continue contraceptive precautions until two consecutive seminal specimens, taken at intervals of 2–4 weeks, are both negative. Should sperms in large numbers continue to appear, it is advisable to re-explore the scrotum under general anaesthesia, so as to allow more thorough examination, to exclude re-canalization of one vas, or a failure at the original operation to identify the vas correctly. The rapidity with which sperm disappear from the semen after vasectomy depends upon the frequency of intercourse—by which, of course, the reservoirs are emptied. It is generally believed that most men require at least ten ejaculations before they have exhausted their stored sperm; and the time taken to achieve this varies greatly with age, pain-tolerance, and virility.

## Vasectomy Counselling

As with the provision of contraception and abortion, sterilization calls for the skills and experience of doctors, but the final decision is with the man or woman concerned. Vasectomy counselling is a well-developed example of the interchange between doctor and client rather than between doctor and patient. It is worth exploring in more detail what each seeks from such an interchange.

At the interview with both partners the doctor wants to make sure that the decision, if taken, will be soundly based and thoroughly considered. All doctors have a fear of iatrogenic (doctor-produced) disease and clearly the psychological ill-effects of sterilization are in this category if it has come to be resented but cannot be reversed. He will try to explore the previous contra-ceptive policy and the reasons why it is now to be changed. He will need to take a careful medical history of both partners and will try to assess something of their relationship and stability. On a sexual plane he will wish to be assured that neither partner is seeking the vasectomy in the hope that it will, of itself, improve sexual gratification or performance.

Despite the provider-client relationship, the doctor by virtue of his knowledge and special skill tends to remain in a position of authority and usually guides the interview. He has an obliga-tion to describe and explain the operation, what it is like when the procedure actually takes place under local anaesthesia and its long-term effects. He is in the difficult position of needing to call attention to all likely ill-effects and complications without pre-senting these in an alarming way. Since the ultimate responsi-bility inevitably lies with the doctor who performs the operation,

84

it is usual for this interview to be conducted by himself, or a member of the same vasectomy team. If such a team exists, it is possible for the couple to discuss their position and decision with a trained social worker or experienced lay-counsellor rather than with a doctor and it is arguable that such an interview is more likely to result in a fair discussion.

During the course of a properly conducted interview there is much personal interaction which will give the counsellor some guidance as to how the couple view the operation and its effects. The potentially vulnerable man should thus be identified, or at least the need for deeper probing to ensure that he will not feel mutilated by the operation.

Most experienced counsellors consider that special caution is indicated where the couple show signs of marital instability or lack of harmony. An obvious situation is one where the husband is being pushed into his vasectomy by a wife who is suffering from an obscure dissatisfaction. Further probing may disclose the underlying motivation of the partners though it must be borne in mind that few marital situations are ever as simple and straightforward as they seem on the surface.

Counselling must include comprehensive instructions about shaving the scrotal area beforehand and the arrangements for follow-up and semen testing. Although the possibility of re-uniting the cut ends of the vas should be discussed, it is essential that the man should be warned that vasectomy may well prove to be irreversible and that it should not be accepted unless he is prepared for it to be permanent.

## Effects on Men

Operations upon the genitals have a primitive symbolism and are frightening to even the most rational. Anthropologists are well aware of the symbolic effects of ritual circumcision in all its forms. The persistence of circumcision, apart from its religious practice, in Western communities where there is no medical indication is in itself a fascinating subject for study.

An operation upon the genital area which deliberately removes fertility can reasonably be expected to have deep psychological connotations. It may well be seen as a threat to a man's potency and might well affect his view of himself as a virile lover. In practice, it seems that acceptors of vasectomy have already over-come these fears if they ever experienced them. Vasectomized men are usually very happy as far as their operation is concerned, as has been established by surveys carried out by the Simon Population Trust and from a smaller but more detailed study by Ziegler and his colleagues of the Scripps Foundation in the U.S.A.[10]

Vasectomized men tend to go around persuading others to have the operation. There are clearly two possible interpretations: either they find the operation such a boon they really want others to share their good fortune, or they feel insecure and threatened following the operation and want the security of sharing the experience with many others. The Scripps study showed that four years after vasectomy there were no demonstrable differences between acceptors and the control group whose partners took oral contraceptive pills.

Wolfers, in a study of almost 100 men vasectomized at a Swindon clinic, found a small number had psycho-sexual problems later, but almost every one of them had a history of sexual difficulty before the operation.[11] It may be that one kind of vulnerability stems from a belief, perhaps covertly held, that the operation will in some magical way improve sexual performance. It is very important that such beliefs should be brought out and discussed at the pre-operative interview.

When a man decides upon vasectomy without being urged by his consort or others he is likely to be satisfied with the operation. Deys has suggested that in those marriages where the man is dominant and makes the major decisions he is more likely to choose a male form of fertility control, such as a condom at first and later vasectomy; and, because he has made the choice, the outcome is likely to be well accepted by both partners.[12]

## Possibility of Reversal

Can a vasectomy be successfully reversed? Hanley claims good results in 30% or more of attempts at re-union.[13] Some Indian surgeons claim a much higher success rate. Restoring continuity of the tube itself is not the only requirement. There seems to be a functional quality that must be restored too, perhaps a propulsive muscular wave of the vasa deferentia, perhaps some biochemical factor. At one time it was thought that antibodies in the man's bloodstream that could cause spermatozoa to clump together were the cause of failure to restore fertility, but these have been shown to reach significant levels in only a small minority of vasectomized men. Such antibodies are certainly commoner in populations of naturally infertile men, so there may be *some* small element of truth in this theory.

Vasectomy is far simpler and safer than any form of female sterilization and the chances of failure are equally remote for sterilization performed on a woman or a man. Also vasectomy is potentially reversible whereas no form of female sterilization can truly be described as such. These are big advantages which should receive due weight when the questions of sterilization and of which partner should be sterilized are discussed. The idea that vasectomy is always preferable to female sterilization is, however, an over-simplification. Each couple with its medical and social problems needs individual counselling, and the partners need to make a choice which is fully acceptable to both partners before it is implemented.

When a couple come seeking sterilization it is usually apparent that one partner is more strongly opposed to further children than the other. Often such a conviction is deeply felt and would survive even the loss of the spouse and ensuing remarriage. In general, it is this partner who will be the less likely to suffer from sterilization, and it is he or she who ideally should be sterilized if all other considerations are equal. The other considerations include past and present health. If the woman is seriously or chronically ill or if she has suffered with illnesses associated with pregnancy so that further childbearing would be hazardous or ill-advised, then it may well be obvious that she is the better candidate for sterilization. At the same time, as with abortion, a paradox exists in that the worse the woman's condition the more likely is her illness to make the operation more dangerous for her. In such a situation the ages of the couple and of the youngest child may be an important factor. If the man is young with young children and his sick wife dies he will probably remarry a wife young enough to want children of her own. Sterilization for him, though medically logical, is better avoided —that is, in just the case where superficially it seems strongly desirable.

87

## Limitations on Use

Until 1972 most men had to pay for vasectomies—either an individual surgeon, or what was usually a smaller fee to an agency such as the Family Planning Association, which ran special vasectomy clinics. During that year the Family Planning (Vasectomy) Act made vasectomy theoretically just as freely available from local authorities in the U.K. as contraceptives. No special provision was made to enable women to be sterilized by choice free of charge, but even by 1972 it had in practice become fairly easy for women living in most parts of the country to obtain sterilization under the N.H.S. if they were willing to accept it immediately after, or with, childbirth or abortion.

Before 1972 it had been difficult for really indigent family men, especially with large families, to find the money for a vasectomy. For this and possibly for other reasons those who took advantage of the arrangements in the agency clinics were mostly skilled manual workers with a reasonable level of prosperity and a well-planned and organized family life. Most had used condoms for previous contraception which might indicate that the man tended to dominate in birth control decisions. Average family size in the King's College Hospital series of vasectomies in South London was 2·71, not very much greater than the norm for that generation of families.[14] The type of man mentioned is gregarious and the 'proselytizing' effect was well shown when clinics found they were dealing with a succession of clients from the same pub, football club, fire station, or police station. This type of 'clustered diffusion', was absolutely characteristic of the spread of vasectomy at that time.

The effects of providing vasectomy everywhere free of charge remain to be seen. At the time of writing the provision of vasectomy varies widely in different parts of the country according to the policies of the local Area Health Authorities. It may be that in the future we shall see vasectomy accepted well by the lower-paid working-class man and immigrant groups.

Age is an important factor in determining who will be refused vasectomy in an average agency clinic. A variety of reasons may be given but relatively young people find difficulty in persuading doctors to agree to sterilization. The obvious reason is that they have a long time ahead in which to change their minds; though on the other hand more unwanted conceptions will be prevented by sterilizing younger people, not only because they have more years in which to produce an unwanted pregnancy, but also because their inherent fertility is higher. Coitus may also be more frequent and the chance of a contraceptive mistake greater—depending on the type of method used.

There is an argument, in other words, for encouraging younger couples to use sterilization if only one could be sure that their family intentions were very firmly decided. More research is needed to determine the merits of such a policy. Only in recent times has vasectomy become utilized by a sufficient number of younger couples for possible ill-effects to become statistically apparent. This difficulty could be avoided if there were methods of sterilization which could be reversed with greater certainty of success.

The young couples who confound sterilization counsellors are the small number who come, sometimes only just engaged, seeking sterilization because they do not believe they will ever want children. If they are both in an older age group—say 35 or older—there is no great problem; but if they are young and have never tried effective contraception, the counsellor will inevitably feel cautious and is unlikely to recommend such an irreversible step. One thing is certain: such a couple tend to get very angry if vasectomy is refused.

There is no doubt of the important part currently played by both female and male sterilization in controlling unwanted fertility at the end of family building, and it is reasonable and desirable that it be more widely used.

## Legal Implications

Sterilization operations are governed by the same legal requirements as any other operation—namely, that the patient should give informed permission for whatever procedure is to be performed. Neither spouse in a marriage has rights over the other's body, and the permission of the spouse is not mandatory prior to sterilization. Nevertheless, deliberately-concealed sterilization by either husband or wife might have legal implications in the dissolution of a marriage. Normally any doctor would seek the permission and agreement of the spouse before performing a sterilizing operation, and virtually all clinics providing such services insist upon signed permission from the spouse. There may be rare occasions when it is desirable to carry out sterilization without awaiting such agreement as, for example, when an emergency operation is performed upon a woman for whom there are strong medical reasons against further childbearing. Sterilization during such an operation may be easy and free of extra risk, whereas to await permission and to perform another operation later might entail extra hazards.

A vexed question is the sterilization of women who are unable to give informed consent. The mentally defective woman, particularly if she has already had one or more abortions, who is unable to take effective contraceptive precautions provides a good example of a strong social indication for sterilization, but informed consent cannot really be obtained. In general this sort of problem is resolved by consultation between the doctor involved and the guardian or parent of the woman, though she should always be told what was proposed. Sterilization of mentally defective girls under the age of sixteen would seem merely to provide a special example of this dilemma. In such cases it is hypocritical to insist that the operation is delayed until the girl is sixteen if it is sure her mental abilities will not have developed and she will not in truth be any better placed to give informed consent. These are essentially social and not medical decisions. They should be decided by the legal guardians with medical advice from whatever specialist may be concerned. The main area of difficulty lies in how sure one can be in predicting her future capabilities.

# References

1. Bone, M., *Family Planning Services in England and Wales*, pp. 20–21. Her Majesty's Stationery Office, London, 1973.
2. Pratt, I. W., quoted in: *International Family Planning Digest*, 1 (2) 7, 1975.
3. Baird, D., *Journal of Biosocial Science*, 7, 77–97, 1975.
4. Muldoon, M. J., *British Medical Journal*, 1, 84, 1972.
5. Keyfitz, N., *Social Biology*, 18, 109–21, 1971.
6. Schofield, M., *The Sexual Behaviour of Young People*, Longmans, London, 1965.
7. Moraes, D., *A Matter of People*, Deutsch, London, 1974.
8. Jackson, L. N., Hanley, H., and Baird, D., *Vasectomy: Follow-Up of 1000 Cases*. Casey, Cambridge, 1969.
9. Waite, M., *British Medical Journal*, 2, 629–34, 1973.
10. Ziegler, F. J., *Annals of Internal Medicine*, 73, 853, 1970.
11. Wolfers, H., *British Medical Journal*, 4, 297–300, 1970.
12. Deys, C. M., *Clinical Proceedings of Medical and Scientific Congress*, International Planned Parenthood Federation, South East Asia and Oceania Region, pp. 187–92. Supplement to Australia and New Zealand Journal of Obstetrics and Gynaecology, 1972.
13. Hanley, H. G., *British Journal of Urology*, 44, 721–22, 1972.
14. McEwan, J., Newton, J., Yates-Bell, A., and Hoy, J., *Contraception*, 9, 177–92, 1974.

# 5 CONCLUSION

## *People, Politics and Education*

CONCEPTION and contraception are not simple opposites. If a couple are having normal sexual relations then conception follows naturally and requires no special planning or action. On the other hand, contraception is voluntary reversible action to prevent pregnancy despite continuing coitus. It may require a single definitive action by one partner, or it may require repeated actions involving both partners to some extent at every sexual act. These premeditated actions characterize the difference between conception and contraceptive behaviour. Family planners emphasize this difference and urge people to practise contraception as a regular routine and take some positive step when a baby is desired, 'planned', or 'wanted'. We need to study the application of these ideas to human fertility patterns and to assess how successful or otherwise the planners have been in their aims.

Shortly after the Second World War scientific writers, in particular Julian Huxley, first called attention to the impending world population crisis. Previously in Western Europe, and especially in Britain and France, there had been considerable anxiety about the decline in fertility that accompanied the lowering of living standards after the Great Depression of the late nineteen-twenties. In those days family planners had urged government provision of a contraceptive service on the grounds that promotion of maternal health by better spacing of babies would achieve an overall increase in births. This is an argument that has not been heard in recent years. Family planners have moved any directive interest they have towards the provision of contraceptive services in order to prevent an undesirable population increase. A world-wide interest in this project has led to a number of social studies on contraceptive behaviour in the United States and in Britain. We now have very solid evidence about correlations of certain social factors with the use of those contraceptive methods usually considered the most effective—

that is, methods requiring professional advice such as the pill, cap and intra-uterine device. These studies show that people failing to use effective contraception tend to be couples of poorer education, lower socio-economic class, and those whose background or religious faith is hostile to 'artificial' contraception. As might be expected, these groups also tend to have larger families.

Before a couple can take contraceptive action they must have passed through certain psychological processes. First, they must know and understand that contraception is possible. However obvious it sounds, this step requires some verbal imagery around which the appropriate thoughts can revolve. Some essential words are very difficult and unlikely to be known by the illiterate who do not receive their information through the written word. There are also linguistic blocks to overcome, particularly where emotional or religious prejudice runs high. The importance of words as names is demonstrated by the fact that in Dublin condoms are still known as 't'ings'—local officialdom has even refused to accept the registered trade name 'Durex'.

Second, poor people cannot always use adequate contraceptive techniques because the most effective methods are the most expensive. But now that the N.H.S. is responsible for the cost of contraception in Britain this will no longer be relevant here.

The third, and possibly the most important reason why the poor, ill-educated, and underprivileged fail to use contraception may well be the need to consult professionals whose authoritarian image inhibits them. It is for this reason that all unnecessary consultations and examinations are positively harmful.

Such difficulties lead to a reconsideration of whether the contraceptive pill should require medical prescription or be made freely available over the counter. In general, the principle followed is that drugs that carry an established risk of death or serious illness are available only on prescription; but many drugs (e.g. aspirin, phenacetin) that have traditionally been freely available remain so even though they are now known to have certain dangers. The pill is analogous to drugs given by midwives on their own responsibility during the management of labour. In the great majority of cases, these drugs are perfectly safe when given by a midwife—she would obtain the advice of a doctor if there were any associated illness for which they might be harmful or if any serious adverse effects arose. It seems quite reasonable therefore that the established oestrogen-progestogen pills should be made available on the prescription of a suitably trained midwife, nurse, or health visitor.[1]

Up to now, there have been no reports of serious adverse effects of the progestogen-only pills which are somewhat less effective against pregnancy than the combined pills, and their free sale 'over the counter' or by mail order would not be dangerous and would make an effective method of contraception available to women who are unwilling to consult a doctor or attend a clinic. Naturally, these progestogen-only pills must remain available from professional sources as well.

The authorities in countries such as Spain will smile at our current preoccupation with this question. By ignoring the contraceptive qualities of the pill in a country where contraception is illegal they have provided a liberal solution. Anyone can buy the pill across the chemist's counter if they have the money.

## Contraception and Family Building

The use or otherwise of contraception is often wrongly associated with the intentions of family building—that is the number and spacing of children. Couples with large families tend to have social factors in their lives similar to those affecting people who have actually failed to use contraception. But it does not follow that a couple with poor education and possibly a Catholic upbringing who had a large family did so because of failure to use contraception: they may well have made a conscious choice.

Family planners often over-estimate the importance of so-called effective techniques. There is increasing evidence that the really important factor is the decision taken by the couple on their desired family size, and that once this decision has been firmly made it tends to be followed through irrespective of the availability of 'effective' contraceptives. This is a very fundamental point. If, for example, a couple are determined to avoid more children, but have learnt only the withdrawal technique, they will nevertheless use this rigidly, never allowing their emotions to over-run their determination, and thereby make withdrawal effective. Such determined couples will resort to abortion, legal or illegal, should pregnancy occur. True effectiveness depends on motivation.

94

The question of genuine motivation is particularly important when considering contraceptive aid to developing countries. Mamdani's commentary on the Khanna Study is revealing. A group of researchers from Harvard studied fertility patterns in two Punjab villages in the 1950s.[2] They then gave one village a liberal supply of foaming vaginal tablets together with intensive educational and motivational training leading to improved economic standards. They compared their fertility pattern with that of the neighbouring village without the contraceptives. Decline in family size and birth-rates were shown over 10 and 15 years. Some years later Mamdani returned to the area and found that after the departure of the researchers, fertility had returned to the traditional high-parity family pattern and that the long-term attitudes had not really changed.[3] He remarked on the traditional hospitality of Khanna villagers to guests, which entailed following the advice and encouragement of the distinguished Americans whilst they were there, but after they had gone returning with some relief to the patterns of their forbears.

This story indicates the limited usefulness of the large-scale 'engineering' type of strategy in fertility-regulating programmes. Such programmes have largely failed. Where the mass provision of contraceptives appears to have been successful it seems likely that there had been current, possibly coincidental, changes in local fertility patterns. A rise in living standards, for example, makes communities seek to preserve their gain by limiting family size. As has been said before, to the very poor another child makes relatively little difference and may provide some insurance for the parents in their old age. It is only when one's standards are high enough to include a promise of future security that people strive to maintain and bequeath such a way of life by family limitation.

In the U.S.A. and in Britain there have been careful sociological studies on unwanted pregnancy but these give no reliable information about previous family intentions because the reaction of the woman and her consort to an unwanted pregnancy is demonstrable only when the woman is actually pregnant. It is difficult for women (or men) to appreciate the unwantedness of pregnancy in the abstract. A large number of women when seeking abortion use the phrase: 'I've always disapproved of abortion really, but . . .'

Many workers have studied women seeking abortion in an attempt to try and determine the factors which led up to this crisis and particularly why there had been a failure of contraception. Beard and co-workers in their study of N.H.S. patients in South London found that genuine ignorance—not only of contraception, but of sexual matters generally—was an important factor.[4] They found also that sexual guilt and psycho-sexual problems contributed to inadequate contraception.

Pearson, in a comparison of young unmarried first conceivers having an abortion or proceeding to term, found that these two groups differed little in contraceptive knowledge and attitudes in the pre-conception period.[5] He did show, however, that those choosing abortion were more likely to have made more positive efforts to get contraceptive advice and they were also less likely to have satisfactory relationships with the putative father.

Pearson's work shows how easily young single girls drift into their first pregnancy and it is reasonable to speculate that the same thing often happens to young married couples. How many really 'want' and 'plan' their first pregnancy? In contraceptive clinics, at least half the pregnancies first reported by clients are 'unplanned', but this, of course, does not imply that the babies are unwelcome by the time they are born.

Until fairly recently it was not technically feasible to 'plan' each pregnancy in the way that family planners urge; but today, if wives deliberately 'come off the pill' or have their intra-uterine device removed by the doctor in order to conceive, it would seem that the resultant babies are highly likely to be 'wanted' babies.

A major problem is accidental pregnancy after the intended family is complete. In the 1967/8 Marriage Survey by the Population Investigation Committee Glass reported that 14% to 20% of all births to married couples were 'accidental' or 'unexpected'.[6] The Registrar-General's *Supplements on Abortion* in England and Wales show that nearly half the abortions are performed on married women and that most were in their 30s with 2–3 children already.[7] These statistics suggest that unwanted pregnancies after an intended family is complete are not uncommon.

Quite apart from this statistical evidence, unwanted conceptions are inevitable because of the relatively poor use-effectiveness of current contraceptives. Keyfitz (see Chapter 4) has calculated that there is a 40% chance of one further pregnancy in couples who have completed their intended families, if using very effective contraception and having 20 years of potential fertility ahead.[8] Such considerations make it necessary to question the effectiveness of contraception alone as a method of fertility control. However, we lack reliable prospective data on family intentions contrasted with final achievements. Peel, in his prospective study of family intentions, has so far followed his couples for only 10 years and cannot yet comment on accidental conceptions after planned family size has been reached.[9]

Askham, in an Aberdeen study of lower-working-class families with more than three children, has shown that often there was no clear intention of wanting a given number.[10] This was in contrast with the behaviour of working-class couples in skilled occupations who had only two children. Mothers in the first group felt that they had a surplus but felt vague about the reasons: 55% of them had more children than they wanted, whereas in the two-child group 56% felt that they had the desired number. 70% in the high parity/low income group 'took things every day as they came' compared with 50–56% in the two-child group. In the poor the advent of another child has less effect than in a more affluent family which, for example, has hire-purchase commitments to meet each month.

The idea of family-building decisions being determined economically has been rejected by some sociologists but it does seem to gain support from the Askham report and also from such studies as the Family Intentions survey of Woolf.[11] Here the respondents, all married, were asked how many children they would have 'supposing they had no particular worries about money'. On average it was almost one child above the intended family size (3·4 compared with 2·5).

Economic motivation may apply in an industrialized society with its greater mass influence and wider choices available to parents on ways to spend money. Parents will often wish to give their children a high standard of living and a good education and so will try to have only a small family. They are more likely to use effective contraception and the mother may supplement the family income by working when the children reach school age.[12]

In a poor community—for example in a developing country—there is likely to be less faith in the outcome of decision-making and planning. Additional children may represent more hands to help with the work and, in the absence of a social security system, the children are the only security such parents have when they are too old to work or disabled. Under these conditions 'unwanted pregnancy' is an irrelevant and meaningless phrase: a woman may need to bear five children to ensure that there will be one male child surviving to support her in her old age.

## Family Planning and Politics

Throughout the world attempts at government control of family size are certain to be resented. Nevertheless, politicians, having assessed their country's need for a larger or smaller population, have always tried to influence its size. The payment of financial inducements such as child allowances to parents is pro-natalist, though once the system has become hallowed by tradition it may be seen as part of a social security system. To reverse the process and impose financial penalties upon over-fecund couples is not generally considered politically viable. There are, though, large industrial housing estates on the outskirts of Bombay where free schooling is provided only for the first two children in a family; and abortion and sterilization are encouraged if the two-child limit is exceeded.

Because the 19th and 20th centuries have seen an enormous improvement in death control without a concomitant rise in birth control, almost all countries face excessive population increases. The problems of the affluent countries are less dramatic than those of developing countries and their politicians are therefore under less pressure to intervene in such a sensitive field. In India and many other developing countries, however, population growth militates against various reforms and attempted improvements in material conditions. When its population is increasing more rapidly than the real wealth of a country, a falling living standard is inevitable. The Indian government cannot escape its responsibility to promote some form of population restriction: the problem is to decide how best this can be achieved.

Poor developing countries therefore face a paradox. The individual couple has little motivation to restrict family size: we have seen how people with no security have large families. But faced with an ever-increasing population, the politicians are unable to improve social conditions or to provide any real social security. The condition is self-perpetuating, a vicious spiral of poverty.

In developing countries with large natural resources—for example, oil-rich Nigeria—it seems possible that, if these resources were efficiently mobilized, a real rise in living standards and provision of some form of social security would remove the incentive towards excessive fertility. We might then see the rapid development of a stabilized population or, at any rate, a population growth in line with the growth of national wealth.

What is quite certain is that for any national family-planning programme to be successful, the individual couple must be motivated though not dragooned. We have considered economic factors but in this fundamental area of human activity rational considerations may not be paramount. We are all the product of our culture and the radical change in rate of population increase resulting from the increased survival of babies has not yet been reflected in the corresponding cultural changes, which normally take three generations to appear.

The People's Republic of China, with its highly organized and propagated 'Cultural Revolution', seems to have made remarkable progress in population control. Djerassi attributes this success of the Chinese family-planning programme to good organization of pill distribution and a high sense of social discipline.[13] This implies that rapid cultural changes really have in this case been achieved.

Some countries feel the need of more young people for their labour force in order to survive economically: in others, a large national army is thought to be essential.

Dom Moraes has shown how the old slave culture of the African West Coast caused a deep feeling of suspicion against any ideas of birth control originating from the Americans or Europeans.[14] After a visit to Gabon and Senegal he wrote:

'There is a fairly relevant peasant saying in India, in Hindi, "Sarkar mere ma-bap he". This means "the government is my father and my mother" which is what an African or Asian government should be to its multitudes of deprived people and peasants. In Africa, unfortunately, the horrors of the slave trade have branded a mark too deep to be excised for many years to come. It was the white nations which shipped the

99

youth of Africa away, over 300 years, to the Americas. The Arabs started it all, but the Africans now remember the whites more vividly, because they did it on a considerably larger scale. It is now the white nations, perhaps motivated by guilt who are offering family planning to the African countries.

'So to the intellectuals who rule, this offering of a means of controlling population appears suspect. It seems to them another, more devious way of reducing the number of black people in the world, of keeping them eternally under the economic heel of the whites. They therefore do not exactly refuse it, but keep it at arm's length: they are angry with it, and afraid of it, though they realise it may be necessary. But the people of their countries, mostly the women, not only need it but often ask for it. If a government is the father and mother of its people —a loose definition, but valid in the Third World—it must supply its children with the necessities of life.'

Family planners need to be aware of the problem of this type of political misinterpretation of their aims when they try to promote birth control for people with cultures or psychological backgrounds different from their own. Sir Keith Joseph, when Secretary of State for Health and Social Security in Britain, promoted birth control services for the 'feckless and fecund'—the poor and the problem family, for example—as a distinct programme of social engineering. However unnecessary the words used, the money provided did enable local health agencies to promote free and domiciliary contraceptive services for many people in need. Unfortunately and probably unjustly a directed service usually has an unpleasant aura because it is seen as a deliberate attempt to reduce the breeding of one particular social group. This is how the black Africans see the efforts of the Western birth-controllers, and how those of the White South African government are seen by its own black population. The South African government is devoting enormous resources and manpower to the development of contraceptive services directed at the Bantu peoples which make up 82% of the total population and who tend to have large families and a consequently high population growth rate. The liberal observer is comforted by the thought that there are many advantages both to health and to individual comfort from the provision of these contraceptive services, but politically the scheme is liable to founder in the long term because of its apparently racist philosophy.

Similar arguments apply to the provision of international aid for birth control to developing countries. American experts see a threat in the population increase of the Third World, and the United States has been prepared to pour very large sums into birth control schemes to counter this. It would perhaps be more realistic for Western Nations to provide economic and technical aid to Third World countries with the *primary* aim of increasing living standards rather than reducing fertility. Demographic change will follow, but fertility will not become limited voluntarily simply because modern contraception is provided, even if free.

Many Western writers have urged aid to the Third World for reasons it finds suspect. Possibly the clearest of these arguments is that put forward by Garrett Hardin and quoted by Barry Commoner in *The Closing Circle*:[15]

'Every day we [i.e., Americans] are a smaller minority. We are increasing at only one per cent a year; the rest of the world increases twice as fast. By the year 2000 one person in 24 will be an American; in one hundred years only one in 46. If the world is one great commons, in which all food is shared equally, then we are lost. Those who breed faster will replace the rest. In the absence of breeding control, a policy of "one mouth one meal" ultimately produces one totally miserable world. In a less perfect world, the allocation of rights based on territory must be defended if a ruinous breeding race is to be avoided. It is unlikely that civilisation and dignity can survive everywhere; but better in a few places than in none. Fortunate minorities must act as the trustees of a civilization that is threatened by uninformed good intentions'.

Commoner rightly remarks: 'Here only faintly masked is barbarism'. One wonders what can be called civilized or dignified about the attitudes of such hypothetical 'fortunate minorities' in their defended territory. There is probably more civilization and dignity to be found in the back streets of Hong Kong or in the dark huts of a prison camp. Indeed, that kind of statement is a development from Malthus' population theory combined with

Darwin's theory of natural selection. It presupposes a terrible struggle between men of different creeds with no hope of effecting any change in the conditions of life for the Third World.

Liberal Westerners feel bound to support the international promotion of birth control because it seems the only logical course. But one can see that those who are on the receiving end may look twice at a gift that seems to benefit the donor at least as much as the recipient. The gift will come to be wholly acceptable only when it is clear that its value and use is part of a wider programme for raising living standards.

Dom Moraes, the Indian poet and novelist, to whose report we have already referred, was sent round the world by the United Nations Fund for Population Activities to make a qualitative assessment of population problems in human rather than statistical terms, and he brings the reader into human contact with people from widely different cultures, all expressing a common language of suffering and having common feelings related to sex and reproduction.[14] In this emotive and subjective work it is possible to get one man's view of the real effects of religion, tradition and history on human family life. One feels the horror of dirty abortions on a mass scale in the South American countries. One feels the dilemma of humanitarian Catholics trying to reconcile their compassion for the people's struggle against hyperfertility with the absurd and unrealistic pontifications of the Holy See. One can feel the influence of male 'machismo' carried by the Conquistadors (surely a group with a self-selecting bias) from Latin Europe to the mixed multitudes of their heritage. One can also share the depression of the intellectual Gabonese who feel that the future holds little for their infecund people and the courageous, unflagging enthusiasm of the Indian sterilizers in the face of hopeless and ever-increasing congestion. These form the world realities of birth control and are part of the struggle of people to survive outside Hardin's privileged enclave.

## The Future

What are the lessons for the Western World? Firstly, to discard any optimism that birth control alone will be acceptable and effective in the Third World. We shall need to give up much of our national wealth; and this, if on a scale large enough to be effective, will need completely new attitudes, both politically and in our standards of life as individuals. Next we must attempt to put our own house in order. We in the West have not yet achieved genuine birth control, but we must; not only because an unwanted Western baby will consume much more of limited resources, but also because we must present a credible image if we wish to promote the cause of fertility control to others. It is absurd for us to perpetuate inhibitions in the full provision of birth control to all sections of our society. We need, for example, to deal with problems such as the reluctance experienced by many of our people in consulting doctors about contraception.

Thirdly, we must concentrate on education in sexual matters generally and try to make acceptable the idea that sex is for enjoyment and the deepening of mutual relationships. We must attempt to do away with moralist hang-ups and the psychological inhibitions that prevent so many people from achieving their full sexual potential—and that incidentally prevent many from using adequate contraception. We should try to use our sociological expertise in order to help solve the complex problems associated with our new-found ability to separate sex from reproduction. By examining the extent to which our own cultural attitudes towards sex have become outmoded, we should be in a better position to advise and help others whose problems are also primarily cultural.

## Problems of Young People: Pregnancy and Contraception

Medical sociologists and gynaecologists have recently become interested in teenage pregnancy, partly because of the medical, psychological, and social problems involved in these pregnancies, but also because of a developing belief that we are dealing here with some highly informative aspects of reproductive behaviour.

We already know a good deal about the mechanics of reproduction, but we remain woefully ignorant of its emotional and psychological elements. Teenagers probably behave in a similar though less complicated way than adults, so study of teenage conceptions, wanted and unwanted, may be rewarding. In practice relatively few teenage pregnancies can honestly be described as planned and in most cases it seems likely that something has gone badly astray in the decision-making process.

Pregnancy is an outward sign of active sexuality. A married couple show pride in the wife's bulging tummy and this public expression of their coital success is socially acceptable. Perhaps this is why people react so dramatically to teenage pregnancies, which are considered an indication of the moral decadence of our 'permissive' society. It is the sexuality revealed by pregnancy that activates puritanical zeal. Clinical experience shows that although relationships between the unmarried may be deeply felt emotionally, coital frequencies are far less than for an average young married couple.[16] Often the unmarried young can make love only in difficult or congested circumstances—factors which mitigate against the development of full sexual enjoyment. Housing is a major problem for young lovers wanting to live together.

Schofield's follow-up study in 1972 showed how common sex problems were in the young and sexually active.[17] Only 43% felt they had no problem about sex and many were anxious because they felt their sexual performance or experience was not as good as it ought to be. A surprising number (16% of boys and 9% of girls) reported guilt feelings. At the time of this survey, only 7% of respondents had not had coital experience. The sample indicated that by the age of eighteen 34% of the boys and 17% of the girls were sexually experienced.

Contraception tends not to be used effectively by young teenagers (according to Schofield's first survey in 1965) and pregnant teenagers illustrate this point.[18] The fact that young teenage pregnancies are not very common suggests either that there is a high proportion of infertile girls at this age or that coital activity is not common among those under 16. The menarche is gradually moving to an earlier age in Western Europe, but the average length of time from the commencement of menstruation to full fertility is not precisely known. If the menarche is at 12 years of age, it would be reasonable to assume full fertility by 14.

We have reliable data from the Registrar-General's *Supplements on Abortion* of the proportion of young teenage girls in England and Wales who have legal terminations of pregnancy. In all areas abortions for these girls are usually much more easily obtained under the National Health Service than for other age groups. 61% of legal abortions in girls under the age of 16 were performed in N.H.S. hospitals in 1973 as against 50% for all resident women having such abortions. Table 1 shows that the proportion of abortions involving young teenagers is small.

*Table 1*

*Legal Abortions in Young Teenagers: England and Wales residents, 1970–73*

| | Numbers | | Percentage of all Abortions | |
| | Under 15 | Aged 15 | Under 15 | Aged 15 |
|---|---|---|---|---|
| 1970 | 499 | 1,233 | 0·7 | 1·6 |
| 1971 | 625 | 1,671 | 0·7 | 1·8 |
| 1972 | 691 | 2,113 | 0·6 | 1·9 |
| 1973 | 820 | 2,270 | 0·7 | 2·1 |

During a five-month period at King's College Hospital, London, which serves a district of 260,000 people, 54 pregnant girls of under 17 were seen and 29 of them requested an abortion. It has been suggested that West Indian girls accept teenage child-bearing as a normal event, but 10 out of 13 pregnant West Indian girls under 17 wanted abortion.[16]

In spite of the comparatively small size of the problem of pregnancy and of active sexuality in young teenagers some medical authorities list a fearsome series of hypothetical pathological processes that may affect the girls in question including obstetric disasters, permanent ill-health, gonorrhoea, uterine cancer, permanent infertility, recurring miscarriages, etc.

Pregnancy and childbirth in the very young does carry a greater risk for the baby, but this is a situation with which modern obstetric care should be able to cope.[19] One element in the problem is behavioural and possibly legal in that many of these young girls continuing with a pregnancy wait until late gestation before first attending an antenatal clinic. Many are under the impression that their boyfriends will be in trouble if they go to hospital pregnant under the age of 16. Others like to be married before they first attend. In both cases social pressures—real or imaginary —mitigate against good obstetric care.

It is difficult to see where the medical Jeremiahs find evidence for the other disasters they fear. Recurrent miscarriages can occur if the neck of the womb is damaged in an abortion though, with modern methods such as the thin plastic Karman cannula, this is very unlikely to occur. A greater risk of cancer of the uterine cervix is statistically associated with increased exposure to coitus, but whether this would have a serious effect if first coitus was at 14 instead of 18 is doubtful.[20] In any case the frequency of intercourse is low in young teenagers. It has been suggested that having multiple partners increases the cancer risk, but we have no evidence that the under-17s are more prone to have multiple partners than anyone else.

What about gonorrhoea? There was an alarming rise in notified gonorrhoea between 1968 and 1971 followed by a recession in 1972. The proportion among the under 16s however was very small, viz.:

*Table 2*

*New Cases of Gonorrhoea per 100,000 Population by Age seen at Hospital Clinics in England* [21]

| Age | 1968 | 1969 | 1970 | 1971 | 1972 | 1973 |
|---|---|---|---|---|---|---|
| Under 16 | 2·7 | 3·7 | 4·1 | 4·5 | 4·5 | 5·2 |
| 20–24 | 411·1 | 459·0 | 488·5 | 527·5 | 535·4 | 602·4 |
| All ages | 95·6 | 108·3 | 115·7 | 121·3 | 115·3 | 126·1 |

Involuntary sterility can occur from gonorrhoeal infection and from Fallopian tube inflammation following abortion, but the number of cases must be minute in girls under the age of 16. Infection following abortion is very much less of a danger when modern methods are used and proper follow-up care is given. Should it occur, the condition is usually completely curable by antibiotics. One medical professor has invoked contraceptive methods as a cause of permanent sterility in the young —the intra-uterine device because of tubal inflammation and the pill by permanently stopping ovulation. There is some doubt whether this last does, in fact, happen to women who use the pill—if so it is in less than 0·5% of users. Low grade tubal inflammation can occur in about 1% of I.U.D. users, but with proper medical care the condition quickly clears up and there is no evidence that any insignificant proportion of I.U.D. users subsequently become sterile.

Medical authorities have contributed to puritanical reactions over 'permissiveness' by fomenting public anxieties about medical conditions that might theoretically arise. As far as teenage sexuality is concerned, the public reaction may simply be an expression of communal guilt, and doctors should concentrate on giving youngsters good and careful treatment: if this is done, teenagers are unlikely to suffer more ill-effects from sex, pregnancy, and childbirth than any other age group.

There may be a failure of professional standards in this field due to emotional problems in the doctor, and the low usage of contraception by young teenagers illustrates the point. Doctors have been reluctant to offer contraception to the very young and have all too often rebuffed them or given them moral lectures when contraceptive advice was wanted. Some doctors have been worried that they might be accused of breaking the law, even though contraception is a measure to prevent pregnancy and, of itself, does not aid or abet unlawful sexual intercourse.

When a doctor believes a girl to be sexually active then the medical defence agencies now advise that he can legally give contraceptive advice irrespective of her age. An action brought before the General Medical Council has established that no doctor should disclose to parents or others that any of his patients of under sixteen are having sexual intercourse, unless he has his patient's permission to do so.

Most of the so-called medical problems of teenage sexuality are largely figments of moralistic imagination, but social problems cannot be dismissed in the same way. Social support for young people when they have babies is inadequate, so it is not surprising that many are poor parents and the marriages, often forced on them by the pregnancy, do not last very long. A high proportion lead to early separation or divorce.

The single girl who has a baby whom she rears herself has a very difficult life. She may be willing to take a job, but is likely to find it difficult to have her child looked after adequately during the day. Many continue at a subsistence level—on Supplementary Benefit from the State. She may prefer to have the baby adopted, but giving up a child is a traumatic experience; or she may apply for a legal abortion, which, though it relieves the problem quickly and safely, is an unpleasant experience and is only a less painful solution to an extremely painful dilemma.

What an abortion may do, however, is to bring the girl's fertility problem to the attention of her medical adviser who may then give her effective contraceptive advice. This is surely the solution to the whole quasi-medico-social problem of teenage sexuality. Few of those who are sexually active want to have a baby. Everything possible should be done to disseminate contraceptive information and describe the availability of contraceptive methods to young people. Most of the under-16s will not be sexually active anyway and will not feel ready for that kind of relationship. Nevertheless, all young people should receive a full account of contraceptive practice as part of essential sex education so that they will appreciate the ethical idea that parenthood should result from a responsible decision and not simply occur by accident.

This is not to say that sex should be taught as an act designed primarily for reproduction. It is, and should be, thought of as being an expression of love between two human beings. Probably in the lifetime of each individual the connection with reproduction will arise in less than 1% of total coital activity, the other 99% being for expressing and communicating emotion.

## Education in Sex and Fertility

Frequently an unwanted pregnancy, due to failure to use effective contraception, reveals the confusion, ignorance, and prejudice-induced psychological blocks which led to the failure. A great deal of attention has been given to the problem by many caring agencies and individuals, and now there is fairly general agreement on the need for better and more broadly based education on all sexual matters, particularly on contraception.

Is it justified and realistic to put one's faith in the educational approach? We have no positive evidence that education is effective. On the other hand we have seen that what is needed is a change in behaviour associated with improved factual knowledge. Educational methods are the only reasonable means we know of effecting such changes. Evaluation is essential at every stage so future policy should be to carry out trials of different methods with repeated attempts to measure their effectiveness.

Schofield and others have shown that friends and contemporaries are a much more important source of information about sex than parents and teachers.[18] The accuracy of such information may be very poor. Since we are well aware that ignorance and irrational bias are important factors in sexual problems, logically we ought at least to try and provide more professional sources of information.

Reporting on a Family Planning Association project in South London, Barnard and McEwan wrote:[22]

'The changes caused by education tend to be permanent. The educated individual makes his own decisions and acts on them according to his own preconceived policy. He does not require his responses to be reinforced by posters or television flashes from time to time. Education in other words, leads to conscious individual responsibility. This is the very essence of the "planned parenthood" philosophy'.

This project was an attempt to graft a family planning element on to sex education schemes. Unfortunately much of the effort over two years was spent in trying to persuade education authorities to start sex education schemes in the first place, let alone to modify them by including a contraceptive element. Then, as now, sex education in South London schools, as in most other places, is practically non-existent.

Dallas, of King's College, London University, is less pessimistic in her comprehensive review and commentary on 'Sex Education in School and Society'.[23] She writes in her foreword '. . . it does exist but on the whole prefers to shun publicity and sensational comment from superficial appraisers'. She mentions work at some individual schools. There are islands of excellence with good implementation of programmes, such as those promoted by the Gloucestershire Education Authority.

The feeling of non-existence, or rather non-impact, comes from an overall view such as national samples like those of the Schofield studies in which the effect of organized sex education could not be detected.[17, 18] This is confirmed by Cartwright's work and appeared in the study at King's College Hospital. It is too early yet to compare those areas where sex education has been provided with the others.

## Sex Education and Teachers

One of the difficulties in developing sex education systems in schools is that this work is outside the normal educational curriculum relating to public examinations. It is therefore not under any form of control by an education authority, but like all 'extracurricular' subjects is provided solely at the discretion of the head teacher of any state school. There is no agreement and certainly no formal guidance as to the time that should be devoted to the project and no special staff establishment for such activities.

Like their medical colleagues, many teachers have difficulties in discussing sex and some actually believe that sex education is harmful: large numbers of teachers feel inadequately trained and inexperienced. Parents seldom ask for sex education to be provided, though the majority welcome such a service when it is available.[24] Teachers and parents whose rigid convictions are bitterly opposed to sex education are usually the most vocal and therefore wield a disproportionate influence upon head teachers, though not on those who are already convinced of the value of sex education. Until sex education is widely acceptable, therefore, we shall lack trained teachers; but at the same time the subject is unlikely to gain acceptance until we have trained staff to teach it.

For those teachers willing to tackle this subject there are various organizations providing a range of aids. The B.B.C. and Grampian T.V. have both produced sensitive audio-visual material. The Stenhouse Schools Council Humanities Curriculum Project has produced Teachers' Kits on 'Relations between the Sexes' and 'The Family'.[25] These are sheets of pictorial or graphic material which are handed round during a group discussion to stimulate a flow of comments and views from all members of the group. The Nuffield Secondary Biology Curriculum also provides a basis for the biological and humanistic elements. For those who feel that explicit and detailed demonstration of coital techniques form a valid part of sexual education Dr. Martin Cole and his co-workers at the Institute for Sexual Research have made films and other audio-visual aids, which have already been accepted for sixth form use in some schools.

If teachers in a school feel reluctant to teach the subject, perhaps the head teacher should get somebody else for sex education as for other aspects of health education. The Inner London Education Authority has developed a peripatetic unit for primary schools, which comes at the head teacher's request and spends 2–3 days covering the whole school, then moves on to another. The method has apparently worked well. Parents are included in a group meeting on sex education for 8–11 year-olds which are sensitively conducted.

There are many objections, however, to calling in specialist teachers from outside the school. One of the aims of formalized sex education is to show that knowledge of sexual functions and behaviour has to be learnt by study and example like any other skill. If it is apparent that the school's own teachers cannot or will not provide this aspect of education, then the student will believe that it is different from all other learning. On a more mundane level there are the problems of who is to deal with any questions and comments when the experts have moved on. Fundamentally, by opting out of sex education, school teachers are indicating that they themselves are not available to discuss and advise pupils on sexual problems. Research is needed into this sphere so that really effective help can be given, and those teachers who seek training should be encouraged financially and otherwise. Now that the government has decided to pay general practitioners specifically for prescribing contraceptives and also provides them with free additional training, it should be prepared to do something analogous for teachers.

## Underlying Causes of Muddled Sex Education

When faced with highly illogical behaviour at community level, we must look for the root causes of the failure by the community to agree upon a more rational approach. In relation to highly controversial subjects like religion, nationalism, politics and sex, a great deal of irrational behaviour is accepted because norms have not been worked out. In the past religion was, as it logically should have been, the main source of irrationality, and more people have been killed, tortured and persecuted in its name than for any other cause. We are now learning and accepting the need for religious tolerance. Similarly nationalism in an imperialistic sense has been discredited, though national cultural characteristics are cherished and promoted, again with mutual

toleran ce. The British have a valuable tradition of political tolerance at home which has not yet been successfully developed
in the emergent world. Sexual behaviour varies so enormously
between different cultures that it is impossible to generalize, but
within Western society this century has seen a great development
of tolerance towards variations from the accepted norm. Divorce,
illegitimate pregnancy, and homosexuality are now accepted
more easily.

Sex differs in fundamental ways from the other three examples
of irrational behaviour. It is the only one that is a basic biological
drive—the others can be avoided by choice or indifference. Sex
within Western culture is personal and highly secretive; our
friends know only too well our feelings on religion, nationalism
and politics, but it is a very exceptional person who talks openly
and truthfully about his sex life. Despite this few would doubt
the paramount importance of sex as a motivating force. The
success of much advertising is based on it.

Because sexual behaviour is so much an expression of cultural
attitudes, it is inevitable that it should derive primarily from
family example and training. Most thoughtful parents believe
that it is their own responsibility to provide their children with a
grounding in sexual behaviour. Indeed, those parents who feel
most strongly on sexual morality and ethics may deeply resent
the intrusion of others, such as teachers, who attempt to provide
an alternative form of sex education. In this sphere of the relationship between family and state education a comparison with
religion is inevitable. The rights of parents to indoctrinate their
children in the religion of their choice is a cherished and important
part of religious tolerance, and the importance of the school as a
source of religious inspiration has correspondingly declined. Many
parents and many teachers feel that for the school to attempt sex
education at a fundamental level—that is, a level where it im-
pinges upon cultural behaviour—is an infringement of the family
prerogative over the upbringing of children. This assumption by
society of the central importance of the family necessarily entails
that the development of sexual education within the school
framework must be limited. This limitation is likely to be
strongest in middle-class groups as the less articulate may be
confused by the lack of a party line. Parental views on religion,
nationalism and politics are fixed and labelled, being thereby

readily passed on to the children. In the sexual sphere, we live in a time of rapid change and the parents may well be unsure of where they stand; they may therefore be unable to formulate an agreed doctrine for the children.

Having exposed the basic difficulties preventing the establishment of routine sex education of real significance in schools, we must now consider how much common ground exists, and as a consequence what chances there are of worthwhile developments. Most parents would almost certainly welcome factual sex information being given to their children by teachers and others. It is only when the almost inevitable moral and ethical overtones are under discussion that ordinary parents feel that their 'rights' are being threatened and in this respect liberal educators have to accept that liberal views carry just as many moral overtones as highly restrictive views. Liberal educationalists will necessarily be obliged to consider and respect the more conservative attitudes that will be held by many parents.

Teachers, as educators, have the skills to instruct children, not only in factual data, but also in the power of assessment of such data and, hopefully, the ability to make and apply decisions soundly based on facts. None of us can claim to have successfully completed a sexual education and it is obvious that teaching skills of a high order are required even to promote really adequate factual knowledge of sex and its ramifications, leaving aside the moral and ethical overtones of sexual behaviour. The problem is to discover how sex education can be reasonably separated from such overtones and yet remain meaningful.

Any genuine form of sex education should include discussion of masturbation, extra-marital sex and homosexuality as well as contraception and venereal disease. In promoting real discussion on these subjects most teachers would have difficulty in behaving 'neutrally'. Appropriately trained doctors and other experts should perhaps be involved in presenting the biological facts about sex, but it is necessary for emotional reactions to be ventilated within the safety of small groups if there is to be a development of rationalism in forming attitudes. Teachers will have the skills required to manage these groups provided they have been appropriately trained. Other professionals such as doctors helping in this work will also need the awareness such training provides.

Sex education should form an integral part of 'education for growing up', 'education for relationships' or 'education for family life'. These can be branching themes that encourage a whole range of content dealing with sexuality, fertility, family building, childbirth, child care, emotional relationships, home economics; and health education regarding diet, medicines and drugs, smoking and pollution. The courses should start in primary schools where many questions about sex and home life are asked by children needing accurate and comprehensive answers.[26]

For children between the ages of 8–10 there should be more formal classwork in groups of about twelve with and without parental participation. At the secondary level nearly all the work should be done in smaller groups, as in the teens emotional reactions become more important. Films or film-strips are useful for factual elements, but they should always be discussed afterwards in group work. Participation of pupils is also important in forming the syllabus: they should have some freedom both in choosing the topics and the order in which they are taken.

As well as group work, it is important for secondary schools to provide an individual counselling service for pupils who may feel the need for private guidance or information. This sort of opportunity for individual teaching can merge into the emotional-problem counselling that many schools now provide to help children cope with stresses from their community life.[27]

Ambitious though this outline of a possible scheme may appear, it does at least contain enough reinforcement and consolidation of learning processes for a reasonable chance of success. It may seem logistically formidable, but there are individual schools such as Quentin Kynaston in North London, where such a scheme is already in operation.[28]

It could well be a realistic possibility that in such a system health workers and teachers could really help one another with mutual benefit. One of the features of organization in our health, social and educational services in Britain is the rigidity of the lines of administrative demarcation. Here is just one of the many areas in which lines need to be crossed at peripheral level to accomplish objectives that themselves cut across the barriers laid down by the hierarchies. Health education so far produced officially has mainly been simple publicity and literature of the pamphlet type. This has little to do with real learning. In the realm of sex and family planning there are enormous opportunities for adequate educational processes which could make lasting changes in our social organization and eventually benefit our whole community.

# References

1. Smith, M., and Kane, P., *The Pill off Prescription*, Birth Control Trust, London, 1975.
2. Wyon, J. B., and Gordon, J. E., *The Khanna Study*, Harvard University Press, Cambridge, Massachusetts, 1971.
3. Mamdani, M., *The Myth of Population Control*, Monthly Review Press, New York, 1972.
4. Beard, R. W., Belsey, E. M., Lal, S., Lewis, S. C., and Greer, H. S., *British Medical Journal*, 1, 418–21, 1974.
5. Pearson, J. F., *Journal of Biosocial Science*, 5, 453, 1973.
6. Glass, D. V., *Population Studies*, Supplement: Towards a Population Policy for the United Kingdom, p. 21. Population Investigation Committee, London, 1970.
7. Registrar-General's Statistical Reviews. Supplements on Abortion, 1968–1973. Her Majesty's Stationery Office, London.
8. Keyfitz, N., *Social Biology*, 18, 109–21, 1971.
9. Peel, J., *The Hull Family Survey II*, *Journal of Biosocial Science*, 4, 333–46, 1972.
10. Askham, J., *Fertility and Deprivation*, Cambridge University Press, Cambridge. 1975.
11. Woolf, M., *Family Intentions*, Her Majesty's Stationery Office, London, 1971.
12. Hawthorn, G., *Population Policy: a Modern Delusion*, Fabian Society, London, 1973.
13. Djerassi, C., *Studies in Family Planning*, 5, (1), 13–30. Population Council, New York, 1974.
14. Moraes, D., *A Matter of People*, pp. 138–39. Deutsch, London, 1974.
15. Commoner, B., *The Closing Circle*, p. 297. Knopf, New York, 1971. (Quoting Hardin, G., *Science*, 172, 1297.)
16. McEwan J., Owens, C., and Newton, J., *Journal of Biosocial Science*, 6, 357–81, 1974.
17. Schofield, M., *The Sexual Behaviour of Young Adults*, Allen Lane, London, 1973.
18. Schofield, M., *The Sexual Behaviour of Young People*, Longmans, London, 1965.
19. Butler, N. R., and Bonham, D. G., *Perinatal Mortality*, Livingstone, London, 1963.
20. Terris, M., Wilson, F., Smith, H., Sprung, E., and Nelson, J. H., *American Journal of Public Health*, 57, (5), pp. 840–47, 1967. *See also:* Beral, V., *Lancet*, 1, 1037–40, 1974.
21. Chief Medical Officer (1973–74). The State of the Public Health for 1972; and for 1973, Her Majesty's Stationery Office, London.
22. Barnard, D., and McEwan, J., *Towards an Educational Policy in Family Planning*, Family Planning Association, London, 1970.
23. Dallas, D. M., *Sex Education in School and Society*, National Foundation for Educational Research, Windsor, 1972.
24. Gill, D. G., Reid, G. D. B., and Smith, D. M., *Sex Education; Press and Parental Perceptions, Health Education Journal*, March issue, pp. 1–9, 1971.
25. Stenhouse, L., *Humanities Curriculum Project*, Schools Council, Heinemann, London, 1970.
26. Dennis, K. J., *The Future of Health and Sex Education*, Symposium Report, 17 November, pp. 14–18. Organon Laboratories, 1973.
27. Jones, A., *School Counselling in Practice*, Ward Lock, London, 1970.
28. Werring, P., *Sex Education Scheme for a Boys' Comprehensive School*, Conference Report (mimeo). King's College Hospital, London, 1974.

# GLOSSARY OF MEDICAL TERMS

*Abortifacient:* drug or other substance tending to induce an abortion.

*Amniocentesis:* the operation of puncturing the amniotic sac, usually by means of a special needle inserted through the walls of the abdomen and uterus, in order to withdraw some of the fluid contained in the sac.

*Amniotic:* relating to the amnion, the membranous sac (or bag) that encloses the foetus in the uterus.

*Antibody:* substance produced by the body in response to the stimulus of an infection or immunization, and that neutralizes the corresponding substance (antigen) contained in the bacteria or viruses in question. The body's 'learnt' ability to produce the appropriate antibodies is permanent and confers immunity to infections. Antibodies can also be produced in response to the presence in the body of any foreign substance, apart from those produced by germs—for instance, the tissue of a transplanted organ.

*Aseptic:* free of bacteria—as, for instance, in the case of the gowns, instruments, etc. used in an operating theatre.

*Cannula:* a tube introduced into a body cavity for the withdrawal of fluid; being commonly used with a trocar or stylet, which is a rod that fits inside the cannula and, having a sharp tip projecting beyond the end of the cannula, achieves the actual penetration, and is then withdrawn, the cannula being left in position.

*Cervix:* neck or lower end of the uterus (though the term is used for other organs also); of firm, muscular tissue, projecting into the top of the vagina, and normally having a narrow central passage plugged with mucus and leading into the main cavity of the uterus, though this passage can become very much wider in labour or when dilated by a surgeon. It is described as incompetent when, following such dilatation, it fails to close up properly to its normal narrow diameter, but is lax and open instead.

*Chromosomal:* relating to the chromosomes, the discrete, finger-like objects, visible under a high-powered microscope, that are present in the nuclei (central parts) of all cells (in particular, the germ cells) and that carry the genes of heredity (see *genes*).

*Coitus:* sexual intercourse.

*Coitus interruptus:* intercourse not carried to completion because the male withdraws his penis from the vagina before ejaculation (ejection of seminal fluid).

*Conceptus:* the product of conception—i.e. the embryo, foetus, or baby, with the membranes and placenta.

*Curettage:* the process of using a curette, being basically similar, in the case of uterine curettage, to the scraping out of a jar with a spoon.

*Curette:* instrument for scraping material from various parts of the body, in particular the uterus; having a long handle and a head roughly shaped like a small-sized spoon.

*Cytomegalovirus:* Type of virus, particularly affecting infants, the illness produced being characterized by the presence in various parts of the body of swollen cells containing virus material.

*Diathermy:* application of heat to a part of the body with the aid of an electric current; commonly used to refer to the process of so destroying diseased tissue (e.g. warts) or of cutting through tissue.

*Embryo:* see *foetus*.

*Estrogen:* substance, natural or synthetic, having an action in the body like that of the hormone produced by the cells round the developing egg (ovum).

*Fallopian tube:* tube, named after an Italian anatomist, Fallopius, leading from the ovary on each side of the body to the top of the uterus; essentially a passage way along which the egg, fertilized or not, can travel into the cavity of the uterus, and up which sperms can travel to meet and fertilize an egg shed by the ovary.

*Foetus* (or fetus): the product of conception developing in the mother's womb (uterus). Commonly doctors refer to the foetus in its early stages as the embryo.

*Gene:* material, found on a number of sites (or loci) on each chromosome. In the case of the germ cells the genes determine much of the mode of development of the organism that results from their union—e.g. colour of eyes, body build, some mental characteristics, liability to certain diseases: the inherited characteristics, in other words.

*Hepatitis:* inflammation of the liver.

*High-parity:* descriptive of a woman who has borne a large number of children (from 'parous' = having borne children).

*Hormonal:* relating to a hormone, a substance produced by one of the glands of internal secretion (thyroid, ovary, testis, etc.) whose products influence the body's functioning in a variety of ways.

*Hysterectomy:* the operation of removal of the uterus (or womb).

*Iatrogenesis:* Literally 'the process of being caused by a physician'; used especially to refer to illness produced by a physician— as, for example, by a drug he had prescribed.

*Immunological:* relating to the body's state of immunity—that is, its ability, by means of antibodies and in other ways, to deal with material, germs, or even transplant organs that are foreign to it. A desirable type of immune response (say, one useful for rejecting an invading bacterium) may be undesirable if applied, say, to a transplanted kidney.

*Intra-vascular:* inside the cavity of an artery or vein.

*I.U.D.:* *I*ntra-*u*terine *d*evice—a small plastic or metal item in various shapes, intended to be inserted into the cavity of the uterus (or womb), and to be left there for some months or years to act as a contraceptive.

*Laparascope:* tube-like instrument, commonly equipped with light, lenses, and forceps, etc., that can be manipulated by the surgeon using it; introduced into the abdomen through a small cut and giving good access to various abdominal organs.

*Laparotomy:* surgical opening of the abdomen.

*Ligate:* tie off.

*Menarche:* the onset of the monthly, menstrual cycles, in a girl.

*Mendelian:* in accordance with the laws of inheritance propounded in the 19th century by the Abbé Mendel in Austria. These are still valid, though they have been much elaborated in more recent times.

*Metabolites:* substances produced in the course of the body's chemical functioning—for instance, glucose from ordinary sugar, urea from protein foods, or carbon dioxide gas from the 'burning' of any energy-providing food.

*Monitoring:* the process of careful, regular observation of some aspect of bodily or mental functioning—the temperature, the pulse rate, etc.

*Mutation:* sudden change in the nature of some inherited characteristic(s) due to a change in one or more genes. Can occur spontaneously or as a result of excessive exposure to X-rays or other stimuli.

*Oestrogen:* see *estrogen*.

*Oocyte:* those cells in the ovary some of which will eventually develop into ova (eggs).

*Ovulation:* the monthly process in which an ovum matures and is shed from the ovary during a woman's reproductive years.

*Pelvic:* relating to the basin-shaped bony structure (the pelvis) in which the lower abdominal organs (the bladder, uterus, ovaries, and lower bowel) are situated.

*Pessaries:* (1) small medicated objects intended for insertion into the vagina, where they will melt and the medicament they contain will be released and exert its effect; or (2) items made of rubber, plastic, etc., and often ring-shaped, to be inserted into the vagina to support the uterus in cases where the latter is tending to sag downwards (prolapse).

*Pituitary:* one of the endocrine glands (or glands of internal secretion), which, as well as producing hormones of its own, produces substances that control the functioning of the other endocrine glands; located just below the brain.

*Placenta:* flat, round, fleshy organ, fixed to the lining of the uterus during pregnancy and connected to the foetus by the umbilical cord. Nourishment is supplied by the mother to the foetus via the placenta, and waste products of the foetus are removed.

*Progesterone:* hormone produced, after an ovum has been shed from the ovary, by the tissue left at the site it occupied. It is, therefore, produced mainly after ovulation and up to the time of the next menstruation—or, of course, to some extent throughout pregnancy if this should occur. Its function is to prepare the uterine lining for the reception and development of the fertilized ovum.

*Progestogen* (or progestagen): substance having a progesterone-like action.

*Rhesus positive* (or negative): as well as the original ABO blood groups, there are two Rhesus (or Rh) groups in man: Rh positive and Rh negative—people who are positive having a substance (antigen) on their red blood cells that will cause them to be clumped together by the blood serum of a rabbit that has been immunized against the red blood cells of a Rhesus monkey. Most people are Rh positive. The main importance of these groups is that, if some blood from a Rh positive foetus or baby should get into the blood circulation of its Rh negative mother during abortion or labour, the mother's body treats the Rh positive blood cells as it would any other foreign substance and 'learns' to make antibodies against them; so that, if the mother subsequently has another Rh positive baby, her body may produce and transfer to the baby enough of the anti-Rh substances (antibodies) to cause a serious reaction, including jaundice. There are now methods of preventing this sequence of events at one or other stage.

*Septicaemia:* A serious type of infection in which bacteria are actually present in quantity in the blood, and popularly known as 'blood poisoning'; much less common now than before the discovery of sulpha drugs and penicillin.

*Spermicidal:* lethal to the spermatozoa or sperm cells.

*Thrombo-embolism:* the process by which a clot forms inside a blood vessel, and may subsequently break off in whole or in part from the lining of the vessel to form an embolus which then travels along the vessel and perhaps to the heart, eventually blocking a blood vessel too narrow to allow it to pass any further onwards—with all the consequences that may arise as a result of the blood supply to some part of the body being thus cut off.

*Trichomoniasis:* an infection of the vagina due to a small organism, the *Trichomonas*, much bigger than bacteria and equipped with whip-like 'limbs' that make it easily recognizable under the microscope. Men are also often infected, but do not usually have symptoms: women complain of discharge and irritation. A drug given by mouth usually cures the condition.

*Tubal ligation:* A tying-off by a surgeon of the Fallopian tubes so that their cavity is completely blocked.

*Vasa Deferensia:* plural of *vas.* Tubes leading from each side of the testicle which carry the sperm to the prostate gland where it is stored until ejaculation.

# INDEX